3/94

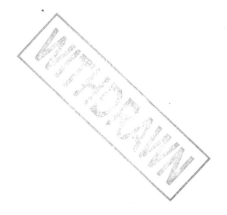

BACR Guidelines for Cardiac Rehabilitation

BACR Guidelines for Cardiac Rehabilitation

Edited by

Andrew J. S. Coats
Hannah M. McGee
Helen C. Stokes
David R. Thompson

on behalf of the British Association for Cardiac Rehabilitation

b

Blackwell
Science

© 1995 by
Blackwell Science Ltd
Editorial Offices:
Osney Mead, Oxford OX2 0EL
25 John Street, London WC1N 2BL
23 Ainslie Place, Edinburgh EH3 6AJ
238 Main Street, Cambridge
  Massachusetts 02142, USA
54 University Street, Carlton
  Victoria 3053, Australia

Other Editorial Offices:
  Arnette Blackwell SA
  1, rue de Lille, 75007 Paris
  France

  Blackwell Wissenschafts-Verlag GmbH
  Kurfürstendamm 57
  10707 Berlin, Germany

  Feldgasse 13, A-1238 Wien
  Austria

First published 1995

Set by DP Photosetting, Aylesbury, Bucks
Set in 10.5 pt Times
Printed and bound in Great Britain
by Hartnolls Ltd, Bodmin, Cornwall

DISTRIBUTORS

Marston Book Services Ltd
PO Box 87
Oxford OX2 0DT
(*Orders*: Tel: 01865 791155
        Fax: 01865 791927
        Telex: 837515)

North America
  Blackwell Science, Inc.
  238 Main Street
  Cambridge, MA 02142
  (*Orders*: Tel: 800 215-1000
          617 876-7000
          Fax: 617 492-5263)

Australia
  Blackwell Science Pty Ltd
  54 University Street
  Carlton, Victoria 3053
  (*Orders*: Tel: 03 347-0300
          Fax: 03 349-3016)

A catalogue record for this title
is available from the British Library

ISBN 0–632–03934–5

Library of Congress
Cataloging-in-Publication Data is available

*'One person with belief
is equal to a force of
ninety-nine who have
only interest'*

John Stuart Mill

This book is dedicated to all those whose belief in the value
of cardiac rehabilitation has made possible the development of the
British Association for Cardiac Rehabilitation.

Contents

List of Contributors

Diane Allaker *MSc*, Health Promotion Specialist (Physical Activity), Health Promotion, High Wycombe.

Jennifer Bell *BA (Hons), MPhil*, Exercise Physiologist, Department of Cardiac Medicine, National Heart and Lung Institute, London.

Hugh Bethell *MB, BChir, MRCP, FRCGP*, Former President, British Association for Cardiac Rehabilitation, Principal in General Practice, Alton Health Centre, Hants.

Andrew J.S. Coats *MA, MB, BChir, FRCP, FRACP, DM, FESC*, Senior Lecturer and Honorary Consultant Cardiologist, Department of Cardiac Medicine, National Heart & Lung Institute, London.

Pat Duff *OBE, BA, RN, RNT*, Independent Nursing Advisor and Trainer.

Amanda Farr *DipCOT, SROT*, Senior Occupational Therapist, Cardiac Rehabilitation Team, Nottingham City Hospital NHS Trust.

Adrianne E. Hardman *MSc, PhD*, Senior Lecturer, Department of Physical Education, Sports Science & Recreation Management, Loughborough University.

Jacqui Lynas *BSc, SRD*, Specialist Lipid Dietician, Cardiac Rehabilitation Team, Conquest Hospital, East Sussex.

Hannah M. McGee *BA (Mod), PhD, RegPsychol, FPsSI, CPsychol, AFBPsS*, Health Psychologist, Department of Cardiology, Beaumont Hospital, Dublin.

Andrew McLeod *BA, MA, MB, BChir, MD, FRCP*, Consultant Cardiologist, Poole Hospital NHS Trust, Dorset.

Helen C. Stokes *RGN*, President, British Association for Cardiac Rehabilitation and Research Fellow, National Institute for Nursing, Radcliffe Infirmary, Oxford.

David R. Thompson *BSc, MA, PhD, RN, FRCN*, Professor of Nursing Studies, Institute of Nursing Studies, University of Hull.

Sally Turner *MCSP, MSc*, District Cardiac Rehabilitation Co-ordinator, The Basingstoke and Alton Cardiac Rehabilitation Unit, Alton, Hants.

Foreword

by Dr Hugh Bethell, Former President of the British Association for Cardiac Rehabilitation, and Helen C. Stokes

The World Health Organization (WHO)'s most recent definition of cardiac rehabilitation (CR)[1] reads as follows:

> The rehabilitation of cardiac patients is the sum of activities required to influence favourably the underlying cause of the disease, as well as the best possible physical, mental and social conditions, so that they may, by their own efforts preserve or resume when lost, as normal a place as possible in the community. Rehabilitation cannot be regarded as an isolated form of therapy but must be integrated with the whole treatment of which it forms only one facet.

It is clear from this brief paragraph that in order to provide a service which may encompass so many factors, a multidiscipinary team of healthcare professionals must be prepared to examine a varied and flexible approach to the provision of CR. The following chapters attempt to portray a historical perspective of the development of CR worldwide, as well as the current position of CR in the UK. Later chapters look at some of the ways in which professionals involved in CR may achieve the provision of service outlined by the WHO above.

Cardiac rehabilitation in the United Kingdom

Cardiac rehabilitation has been slow to develop in the UK. In 1970, a survey of members of the British Cardiac Society identified just nine hospitals which provided some form of exercise programme for cardiac patients. Apart from the work of Dr Lorna Cay at the Astley Ainslie Hospital in Edinburgh, Dr Bernard Groden in Glasgow, and Dr Peter Nixon at the Charing Cross Hospital, London, very little was published in the UK for 10 years. The first large scale controlled trial of CR in the UK was published by Dr Peter Carson and his colleagues in 1982, and subsequently there was a gradual growth in exercise-based cardiac rehabilitation programmes – usually led by nurses or physiotherapists.

In 1987, the Coronary Prevention Group (CPG) held a symposium in London entitled 'Exercise – Heart – Health' with cardiac rehabilitation as one of three main topics. Later that year the CPG set up its Secondary Prevention and Rehabilitation Advisory Committee, under the chairmanship of Dr Hugh Bethell. It's first task was the organization of a national conference 'Recovering From a Heart Attack or Heart Surgery', held in October 1988. This attracted a large audience of health professionals enthusiastic to expand their role in CR and to widen its provision in the UK.

In 1989, the British Heart Foundation (BHF), directed by Professor Desmond Julian, and the Chest, Heart and Stroke Association (CHSA), directed by Sir David Atkinson, joined forces to fund new CR programmes in the UK. Since 1992, the CHSA has changed its involvement in heart disease in England, but remains involved in this area in Scotland and Northen Ireland. As a result of this change, the BHF has continued to provide the funds on its own. Grants of approximately £12 500 per year for two years have been given to ten new centres annually on the understanding that District Health Authorities would take over the funding of the centres at the end of that period. This has resulted in a rapid expansion of the provision of rehabilitation to cardiac patients.

Two reports in recent years[2,3] have documented this development. In 1992, the British Cardiac Society (BCS) published a working party report which included a survey of all the districts in the UK in 1989 and identified 90 CR programmes: 87 in hospitals and 3 community-based. In 1995, a further working group of the BCS published a 1992 survey of CR centres and found that some 74% (161) of district hospitals had such facilities. There was a marked unevenness of provision, however, with deficiencies in London and Wales. The number of patients treated annually was about 23 000, which is approximately 15% of those who might be eligible.

The BCS working party report of 1992 also made recommendations on the setting up and organization of CR programmes – including their educational, psychological and vocational components. It advised that every district hospital in the UK should provide a multidisciplinary, individualized rehabilitation programme for its cardiac patients, paying particular attention to the needs of women and children, and also to ethnic minorities – and to the evaluation of outcomes.

A significant step in the co-ordination of CR throughout the country was the establishment in 1991 of a national newsletter (initiated and edited by Helen Stokes) for programme co-ordinators. Following this, the CPG Secondary Prevention and Rehabilitation Advisory Committee proposed and initiated a national body to represent workers in this field. A working party largely derived from the CPG committee created a constitution for the British Association for Cardiac Rehabilitation (BACR) which held its first meeting in Oxford in September 1992. The aims of this association are to:

■ Promote a greater awareness and understanding of cardiac rehabilitation throughout the healthcare system;

- Facilitate communication and support among multidisciplinary professionals concerned with the rehabilitation of cardiac patients;
- Set national standards for cardiac rehabilitation and monitor the evaluation of these standards;
- Develop training programmes encompassing a multidisciplinary philosophy;
- Promote and facilitate research;
- Liaise with other national and international organizations working in this field.

The BACR has been very active and has grown rapidly in membership. However, there is still a great deal to be done if a high standard of CR service is to be made available to all UK patients who might benefit from it. There must, for example, be a greater willingness for providers to establish comprehensive programmes and for purchasers to pay for them; cardiologists need to become more active and more committed to rehabilitation and to work with programme co-ordinators; there is also a great need for adequate training for CR staff. These guidelines are a start – the first major task which the BACR has undertaken. The guidelines should establish benchmarks against which to develop and evaluate services, and support the activities of professionals and administrators alike in providing a comprehensive service informed by science and evaluated with regard to effectiveness.

1995 sees not only the launch of guidelines for use in the UK, but also the launch of a World Council for Cardiac Rehabilitation. This has stemmed from the fact that there are now formal associations for CR in the USA, Australia, Canada, Europe and South Africa, as well as in the UK, and it is likely that this trend will continue in many other countries around the world. The World Council aims to promote international communication and liaison, to ensure high standards of CR and greater dissemination of research findings.

It is clear that in promoting the implementation and continuing development of these guidelines, and in taking its place in worldwide developments, the British Association for Cardiac Rehabilitation will be busy for many years to come.

References

1. World Health Organization (1993) Needs and Action Priorities in Cardiac Rehabilitation and Secondary Prevention in Patients with Coronary Heart Disease. WHO Technical Report Service 831, WHO Regional Office for Europe, Geneva.
2. Horgan, J., Bethell, H., Carson, P., Davidson, C., Julian, D., Mayou, R. and Nagle, R. (1992) British Cardiac Society Working Party Report on Cardiac Rehabilitation. *British Heart Journal* **67**, 412–8.
3. Davidson, C., Reval, K., Chamberlain, D., Pentecost, B. and Parker, J. (1995) Report of a working group of the British Cardiac Society: cardiac rehabilitation services in the United Kingdom, *British Heart Journal*, **73**, 201–2.

Preface

Cardiac rehabilitation is a rapidly expanding specialty in the United Kingdom (UK). The importance of establishing guidelines for good practice and of maintaining ongoing research and service development is well recognized. The present book has been written and edited by a multidisciplinary team from the British Association for Cardiac Rehabilitation (BACR) to assist this process. It is aimed at all practitioners working in the field. It is not intended as a definitive text, but rather attempts to provide a balanced view of the variety of skills and knowledge which are needed in order to deliver effective and safe rehabilitation services to cardiac patients and their families.

Since cardiac rehabilitation is a rapidly developing service, the issue of standards of practice is of considerable importance. There is widespread agreement about the necessity of having standards in place, but responsibility for their development and implementation is less clear. Patient care can only be enhanced if new knowledge and skills are applied by those with appropriate training and experience. It is imperative that cardiac rehabilitation is demonstrated to be a cost-effective use of limited healthcare resources in an increasingly competitive healthcare climate; this is why research, audit and evaluation are crucial to the development of cardiac rehabilitation services.

This book provides an overview of research findings on cardiac rehabilitation and highlights those areas requiring further investigation or development. It would be an impossible task to include in-depth research coverage of every aspect of cardiac rehabilitation, but it is hoped that the publication will stimulate readers to examine their own practices in the light of current findings and encourage further exploration of relevant issues in their own contexts.

The guidelines for service provision presented here are based on research evidence of effectiveness, and on the current structure for health service delivery in the UK. As a first set of guidelines for the UK, the current recommendations are made in a relatively under-developed service setting. The BACR sees the availability of structured training for professionals as an important complement to published guidelines in the overall aim of improving the availability and standards of cardiac rehabilitation.

The BACR is working jointly with other relevant organizations in the field to develop a programme of education and training which will serve the needs of the multiprofessional group concerned with the delivery of a comprehensive cardiac rehabilitation service. It is anticipated that the next few years will see tremendous strides in development in both the quantity and quality of cardiac rehabilitation services in the UK. It is hoped that the present publication can make a contribution to the achievement of this aspiration.

Andrew J.S. Coats, Hannah M. McGee, Helen C. Stokes, David R. Thompson
on behalf of the British Association for Cardiac Rehabilitation
April 1995

Chapter 1

Historical Background

Summary

This chapter sets out the international history of the scientific development of early mobilization following acute cardiac events, with reference to some of the most significant studies.

Introduction

Exercise as a treatment for heart disease is as old as our knowledge of the condition. Herberden in 1768 noted that his patient with angina pectoris was nearly cured by sawing wood for half an hour per day. However, heart disease was diagnosed infrequently over the next 150 years, and by the time that it was recognized as a serious health problem (early in the twentieth century), the age-old remedy had been forgotten. When a heart attack/myocardial infarction (MI) was diagnosed, prolonged bed rest was thought to be *de rigeur* if the patient's life was to be saved and future assured[1]. It was thought that at least three months was needed to allow the injured zone of the heart's myocardium to be replaced by scar tissue firm enough to support even gentle exercise, and that excessive exertion during this time could lead to rupture of the heart, aneurysm formation, heart failure or even fatal arrhythmias.

> For acute myocardial infarction such rest should be more or less complete for a few weeks; ... careful rest for weeks or months (a minimum of three or four weeks) should be prescribed in order to ensure as sound a healing of the myocardial infarct as possible, with a very gradual and careful convalescence (a minimum of one month after completing the rest period).[2]

As recently as 1968, Davidson's textbook[3] advises:

> ... the duration of rest in bed will naturally depend on the severity of the infarction. Three weeks should be the average period, but after a small infarct, sitting in a chair

should be allowed after about 10 days, and six weeks or more in bed may be necessary after a large infarction, or if cardiac failure has developed.

Doctors and nurses often went to great trouble to keep patients at absolute rest, spoon-feeding them, shaving them and, of course, insisting on the use of the bedpan. The illogicality of the use of the latter was demonstrated by Benton *et al.* in 1950[4]. In an amusing experiment comparing simulated use of the bedpan and the bedside commode they showed a 50% higher oxygen consumption with the former. In absolute terms, the commode demands an oxygen use of about 11.5 ml/min/kg, while the bedpan requires about 16.5 ml/min/kg[5].

Scientific evaluation of early mobilization following cardiac events

In 1944, Dock[6] wrote an article entitled: 'The Evil Sequelae of Complete Bed Rest' in which he catalogued the psychological and physical ill-effects of this treatment.

> The physician must always consider complete bed rest as a highly unphysiologic and definitely hazardous form of therapy.

In 1952, Newman and colleagues[7] noted the deconditioning, boredom and depression produced by prolonged bed rest, together with anxiety when the patient was eventually mobilized. They reported a programme of supervised, increasing activity in hospital, allowing the post-infarct patient to sit on the edge of the bed by the third week, walk a little by the fourth and climb a few stairs before discharge after six weeks. The predominant attitude, however, was still extremely restrictive:

> On occasion a patient, because of insufficient insight, may consider the conservative, slowly progressive activity as ridiculous, and may resent the close supervision.

In the same year Levine and Lown[8] reported their 'armchair' treatment of coronary thrombosis, which was aimed at averting some of the haemodynamic disadvantages of lying flat, with increased venous pressure and venous return leading to 'augmented volume work for the heart'. They observed patients with acute coronary thrombosis who were becoming worse – despite all known measures – and who then benefited immediately and remarkably after being placed in a chair. They got most of their patients out of bed and into an armchair within two days of admission, allowed them to take a few steps by the end of the third week and sent them home after four weeks. They also allowed patients to do more for themselves at an early stage:

> Nearly all patients fed themselves and were either permitted the bedside commode or granted toilet facilities.

One patient who had been kept in bed for eight weeks after an infarct a few months previously, exclaimed: 'What a happier time I had with this attack!' Levine and Lown also noted the probable benefit of their regime in reducing such harmful sequelae of bed rest as constipation, thrombophlebitis, osteoporosis, negative nitrogen balance, hypostatic pneumonia, atelectasis and prostatic difficulties.

This move to early mobilization was not quickly adopted in all quarters, and as recently as 1969, a three week period of bed rest after myocardial infarction was usual practice in this country. In 1971, Harpur and colleagues[9] performed a controlled trial of mobilization comparing 7 days to 21 days and found no difference in cardiac mortality or morbidity, congestive cardiac failure, arrhythmias or aneurysm formation between the two groups. Several further studies have supported these findings[10–13], but these trials have been criticized on the grounds that the patients who were rested longer tended to be the sicker, and that, in any event, the comparisons were between prolonged and very prolonged bed rest!

The policy of early mobilization has not been without its critics. Miller[14] argued that since the removal of necrotic cardiac muscle was not complete before the end of the fourth week, and since collateral circulation is slow to develop, the myocardium may still be at risk if the patient is exercised too early. He recommends that patients should not be discharged less than three weeks after an acute myocardial infarction (AMI). As recently as 1983, Evans[15] strongly criticized the advocates of early mobilization, claiming that the known pathological process demands as much rest as possible during the first few weeks after infarction. He argues that the trials of early versus late mobilization have used too few patients and followed them for too short a period, to demonstrate the increase in complications and mortality which might occur with activity too soon after the attack. His preferred regime is two weeks' rest on anticoagulants, discharge from hospital after three weeks and no strenuous exercise for two to three months. Some backing for this approach has come from an understanding of the remodelling of the left ventricle which is seen particularly in patients with large anterior Q-wave infarctions[16]. This process may be aggravated by too much exercise too soon after the attack[17].

Most clinicians, however, support early mobilization. Over the past ten years many such programmes have been described, usually getting the patient up within two to four days and home within 10–14 days in the uncomplicated cases[18,19] with no obvious detriment and some clear benefits to the patient.

> It is clear that rapid mobilisation and early discharge after myocardial infarction should now be standard practice, and there is no need of further evidence of its safety.

So reported Thornley and Turner in 1977[20]. An even shorter hospital stay has been proposed for low-risk patients by Topol *et al.* in 1988[21]. They randomized 80 patients without complications or early exercise test abnormalities (out of 507 consecutive admissions) to discharge at 3 or at 7–10 days. Follow-up revealed no differences in the outcome for the two groups.

It is a feature of many programmes that they include exercise for the patient while still in hospital as the first stage of rehabilitation. In 1976, Johnston et al.[18] started their patients on calisthenic exercises two days after AMI and included recreational activities, together with education on smoking, diet and future activities. Showing patients that their future will not include a reduction in previous physical activities, and encouraging them to resolve to increase (or maintain, where appropriate) physical fitness, are powerful antidotes to the very common infarct-related depression. This is also the time to involve the patient's family in health education. At discharge, patients should be provided with a detailed instruction sheet on future activities, including advice about home exercise regimes. In 1977, after discharge at two weeks, Thornley and Turner[20] recommended a further two weeks in a convalescent hospital undergoing supervised active rehabilitation and progressive walking. Inpatient exercise programmes to diminish the deconditioning effects of being in hospital have, however, failed to show any benefit[22].

In order to extend the supervision of early exercise and ensure its safety, Harrington et al.[19] in 1981 devised a programme of early mobilization with monitoring. Initially the patient is monitored by electrocardiograph telemetry while washing, shaving, dressing etc., and if this is completed without problems, the patient is then monitored continuously for 24 hours with a portable tape-recorder to detect any arrhythmias and to relate them, if possible, to specific activities. A week or more after the AMI a low level exercise test on a treadmill is used to detect arrhythmias, ischaemia, hypertension or signs of heart failure before starting the patient on a graded exercise programme. Prior to discharge, and again shortly after discharge, the patient is monitored while performing customary home activities.

Many other inpatient programmes now include exercise testing before discharge. This is usually a submaximal test to a heart rate of 120[23,24] unless limited by symptoms at a lower heart rate. A few cardiac units perform maximum or symptom-limited tests[25,26] but this has been criticized as being unnecessarily dangerous. The main benefits of the low-level pre-discharge exercise test include the detection of angina, breathlessness, arrhythmias and hypertension with effort, so that knowledgeable advice can be given to the patient about safe levels of exercise after discharge, and decisions about future management. De Busk and Dennis[27] have pointed out, however, that this information is better gleaned from a three week post-infarct test, which is superior for 'distinguishing high risk from low risk patients and for providing guidelines for the resumption of customary activities in the first month or two after AMI'. For the patient, though, and his or her spouse, the boost in morale given by the demonstration of a reasonable exercise tolerance before discharge from hospital can be very worthwhile.

Early exercise programmes

The harmful effects of AMI and of its treatment on both the physical and the psychological health of the patient, have long been recognized. The first rehabilitation programmes were aimed at helping the patient overcome the psychological ill-effects of the attack and adapt to the prospect of future incapacity. When exercise was performed it was applied during the lengthy hospital stay and was gentle, calisthenic and unlikely to have any effect on cardiovascular performance or improve measurable physical fitness[7,28–30].

In 1954, Chapman and Fraser[31] performed treadmill exercise tests with haemodynamic measurements on nine asymptomatic men with healed myocardial infarction, and compared them with 12 normal controls of the same age group. The patients and controls had similar increases in cardiac output with exercise, but the patients developed higher heart rates, probably because of the deconditioning effect of their prolonged inactivity. The authors commented that their results provided no support for the traditional management of some patients, many of whom 'were required to live a bed-chair, and often miserable, existence after recovery'. Exercise was shown to be safe for the post-infarction patient, and two other factors may have played a part in stimulating the use of physical training in their treatment. The first was the demonstration that physical activity was important in the primary prevention of coronary heart disease (CHD)[32,33]. It was possible, therefore, that exercise might have a secondary preventive role, i.e. by having formerly inactive cardiac patients take exercise, their chances of re-infarction might be reduced. The second factor supporting this hypothesis was the work of Eckstein[34], whose experiments on dogs submitted to coronary artery narrowing indicated that they developed collateral vessels to bypass their narrowed arteries more rapidly if they underwent physical training than if they remained inactive.

In the late 1950s and the 1960s a number of groups in different parts of the world started programmes of exercise training for patients with CHD, and began investigating the results. Israel was the cradle of the large scale rehabilitation effort. As early as 1955, Gottheiner[35] started his clinic for training cardiac patients, and by 1968 had experience of 1,103 patients who had trained for at least five years. After several months of preparatory build-up exercises they graduated to endurance exercises such as running, swimming and cycling, and ultimately the fittest took part in competitive games. Once enrolled, the patients were encouraged to stay in the programme forever. Although there were no strictly comparable controls, Gottheiner felt that the mortality of his group (3.6% over five years) was significantly lower than expected (12%). Also in Israel, Kellerman *et al.*[36] reported the results of physical training of 70 cardiac patients, some as inpatients and some as outpatients. They used a four-month course of working activities, such as gardening, together with gradually increasing gymnasium exercise. The physical working capacity measured on a bicycle ergometer greatly improved in both groups, and the aim of the treatment was usually achieved, that is, to return the patient to work – after, in some cases, a prolonged absence because of post-infarction 'ill-health'. Again from Israel, Brunner[37] observed that cardiac mortality was 'about four times higher in clerks and office workers than in people whose occupations are associated with physical effort'. He accepted patients into a reconditioning course some three months after the AMI, and trained them two or three times weekly with calisthenics, gymnastics and games. He reported the first three years' experience of more than 200 patients, many of whom became fitter than before their AMI and fitter even than non-trained, healthy individuals of the same age. Angina was reduced, even when S–T-segment depression on exercise still occurred. This last point was also noted by Zohman and Tobis[38] in New York. They trained 18 patients by supine bicycling for six weeks at a level just below their angina threshold. Post-training testing showed an improvement in exercise tolerance in six patients, and during a placebo period of six weeks' breathing compressed air, they retained this gain despite ECG deterioration in three cases. They concluded that alongside the peripheral training effect, the psychological benefit was an important component of their patients' improvement.

In Cleveland, Ohio, Hellerstein and his colleagues developed a comprehensive rehabilitation programme for post-infarct patients. Hellerstein and Ford in 1957[39] laid the foundation for this programme in a lengthy article promoting positive action, explanation and education for these patients, and listing the energy costs of different physical activities at work and at play. In the following decade they reported on their experience with the physical training of a large number of post-infarction patients[40-43]. The idea was to: 'add life to years, and perhaps add years to life' for 'habitually sedentary, lazy, hypokinetic, sloppy, endomesomorphic, overweight males' by a programme of enhanced physical activity. They showed that patients who had recovered from AMI could have their physical fitness improved, exercise ECG changes lessened and psychological status raised by a course of exercises which included: 'calisthenics for strength, run-walk sequences for endurance, and recreational exercise for fun'. The exercises were designed to 'stress' the patient to approximately 60–70% of aerobic capacity, but the physical training was only one part of a comprehensive programme which included improvement in nutrition, attainment of normal body weight, giving up smoking and continuation of gainful employment and normal social life.

Meanwhile, elsewhere in the United States, Canada and Scandanavia, the physiological basis of the benefits produced by training cardiac patients was being investigated. Barry *et al.*[44] in Philadelphia, trained six male patients on a bicycle ergometer for 61 weeks and showed improved physical work capacity in five of the six. Improved capacity was slow to develop in some despite training heart rates of 130 per minute or more. Naughton and his colleagues[45] performed the first controlled trial of exercise in 24 post-infarction patients, though the two groups were not strictly comparable since the exercisers had volunteered for the study. Twelve sedentary healthy controls were also studied. After eight months of competitive games, calisthenics and non-competitive jogging, the twelve exercisers had lower heart rates and lower blood pressures at rest and with exercise, than the two sedentary groups. This exercise programme was also applied to larger numbers of cardiac patients and this group went on to establish comprehensive guidelines for the use of exercise in cardiac rehabilitation[46].

In Canada, Rechnitzer *et al.*[47] expanded the controlled trial by including as controls for the exercising cardiac patients, a group of cardiac patients who met for low intensity exercise, and two groups of healthy individuals, one who exercised and one who did not. The numbers were small, just eight in each group, and the exercising cardiac patients showed a significant improvement in the performance of a battery of muscular endurance tests, while the non-exercisers did not. The same team[48] found a greater change for the good in various personality characteristics in exercising cardiac patients than in the non-exercising cardiac patients and the healthy controls, though the controls and sedentary cardiac groups did show sufficient improvement to indicate that at least part of the psychological benefit of exercise therapy was provided by the group setting in which it took place.

In 1966, Varnauskas and his colleagues[49] reported the results of invasive tests in nine cardiac patients before and after exercise training. They demonstrated a reduced cardiac output and left ventricular work at a given submaximal workload after six weeks of regular cycling on an ergometer. In Helsinki, Frick and Katila[50,51] likewise performed invasive studies on patients before and after training, starting just two to four months after infarction, and found a reduced pulse rate and cardiac output during exercise, and also an enhanced stroke volume and left ventricular function after training. Some of this benefit may have been produced by the spontaneous improvement in myocardial performance as the heart recovered from the infarction. The haemodynamic benefits of physical training were further elucidated by Clausen *et al.*[52] in Copenhagen in 1969. They exercised nine cardiac patients, some with and some without angina, for four to six weeks by interval cycling on an ergometer. After the course the oxygen uptake at a given workload was unchanged, indicating constant mechanical efficiency, but the cardiac output fell for a given oxygen uptake. Heart rate at a given workload was lower, and in some cases stroke volume was higher. A reduction in blood pressure both at rest and during exercise resulted in lower cardiac workload. They also found a reduction in blood flow to exercising muscle after training, and concluded that although enhanced cardiac performance accounted for the improvement in some patients, in others the improvement in physical fitness was brought about by alterations in peripheral circulatory regulation.

Over the past thirty years, there has been a gradual growth in the acceptance world-wide of the benefits of exercise for patients with heart disease and a slow spread of rehabilitation programmes in most Western countries.There has also been a progressive change from exercise-only programmes to multifactorial intervention, as the importance of education, risk factor modification and stress management have been increasingly recognized and evaluated. In most countries, however, there is still a very long way to go before comprehensive rehabilitation for all patients following acute cardiac events can be provided. It is hoped that these guidelines may play a part in achieving this goal in the UK.

References

1. White, P.D. (1951) *Heart Disease*, London: Macmillan Co.
2. Wood, P. (1968) *Diseases of the Heart and Circulation*, London: Eyre & Spottiswoode.
3. Davidson, S. (1968) *The Principles and Practice of Medicine*, Edinburgh: E&S Livingstone Ltd.
4. Benton, J.G., Brown, H. and Rusk, H.A. (1950) Energy expended by patients on the bedpan and bedside commode, *Journal of the American Medical Association*, **44**, 1443–7.
5. Douglas, J.E. and Wilkes, T.D. (1975) Reconditioning cardiac patients, *American Family Physician*, **11**, 123–9.
6. Dock, W. (1944) The evil sequelae of complete bed rest. *Journal of the American Medical Association*, **125**, 1083–5.
7. Newman, L.B., Andrews, M.F., Koblish, M.O. and Barer, L.A. (1952) Physical medicine and rehabilitation in acute myocardial infarction, *Archives of Internal Medicine*, **89**, 552–61.
8. Levine, S.A. and Lown, B. (1952) Armchair treatment of acute coronary thrombosis, *Journal of the American Medical Association*, **148**, 1365–9.
9. Harpur, J.E., Kellett, R.J., Conner, W.T., Galbraith, H.J.B., Hamilton, M., Murray, J.J., Swallow, J.H. and Rose, G.A. (1971) Controlled trial of early mobilisation and discharge from hospital in uncomplicated myocardial infarction, *Lancet*, **ii**, 1331–4.
10. Groden, B.M., Allison, A. and Shaw, G.B. (1967) Management of myocardial infarction. The effect of early mobilisation, *Scottish Medical Journal*, **12**, 435–40.
11. Hayes, M.J., Morris, G.H. and Hampton, J.R. (1974) Comparison of mobilisation after two and nine days in uncomplicated myocardial infarction, *British Medical Journal*, **3**, 10–13.
12. Abraham, A.S., Sever, Y., Weinstein, M., Dollberg, M. and Menczel, J. (1975) Value of early ambulation in patients with and without complications after acute myocardial infarction, *New England Journal of Medicine*, **292**, 719–22.
13. McNeer, J.F., Wallace, A.C., Wagner, G.S., Starmer, C.P. and Rosati, R.A. (1975) The course of acute myocardial infarction. Feasibility of early discharge of the uncomplicated patient, *Circulation*, **51**, 410–3.
14. Miller, A.J. (1976) Rehabilitation and length of hospitalisation after acute myocardial infarction, *American Heart Journal*, **92**, 547–8.
15. Evans, D.W. (1983) Early mobilisation after myocardial infarction, *Journal of the Royal College of Physicians*, **17**, 217–8.

16. Pfeffer, M.A. and Braunwald, E. (1990) Ventricular remodeling after myocardial infarction, *Circulation*, **81**, 1161–72.

17. Jugdutt, B.I., Michorowski, B.L. and Kappagoda, C.T. (1988) Exercise training after anterior Q-wave myocardial infarction: importance of regional left ventricular function and topography, *Journal of the American College of Cardiology*, **12**, 362–72.

18. Johnston, B.L., Cantwell, J.D. and Fletcher, G.F. (1976) Eight steps to inpatient cardiac rehabilitation: the team effort – methodology and preliminary results, *Heart and Lung*, **5**, 97–111.

19. Harrington, K.A., Smith, K.H., Schumacher, M., Lunsford, B.R., Watson, K.L. and Selvester, R.H. (1981) Cardiac rehabilitation: evaluation and intervention less than 6 weeks after myocardial infarction, *Archives of Physical Medicine and Rehabilitation*, **62**, 151–5.

20. Thornley, P.E. and Turner, W.D. (1977) Rapid mobilisation after acute myocardial infarction. First step in rehabilitation and secondary prevention, *British Heart Journal*, **39**, 471–6.

21. Topol, E.J., Burek, K., O'Neill, W., Kewman, D., Kander, N., Shea, M., Schork, M., Kirscht, J., Juni, J. and Pitt, B. (1988) A randomized controlled trial of hospital discharge three days after myocardial infarction in the era of reperfusion, *New England Journal of Medicine*, **318**, 1083–8.

22. Sivarajan, E.S., Bruce, R.A., Almes, M.J., Green, B., Belanger, L., Lindskog, B.D., Newton, K.M. and Mansfield, L.W. (1981) In-hospital exercise after myocardial infarction does not improve treadmill performance, *New England Journal of Medicine*, **305**, 357–62.

23. Ericsson, M., Granath, A., Ohlsen, P., Sodermark, T. and Volpe, U. (1973) Arrhythmias and symptoms during treadmill testing three weeks after myocardial infarction in 100 patients, *British Heart Journal*, **35**, 787–90.

24. Mansfield, L.W., Sivarajan, E.S. and Bruce, R.A. (1978) Exercise testing of myocardial infarction patients prior to hospital discharge: A quantitative basis for exercise prescription, *Cardiac Rehabilitation*, **8**, 17–20.

25. Ibsen, H., Kjoller, E., Styperck, J. and Pedersen, A. (1975) Routine exercise ECG three weeks after acute myocardial infarction, *Acta Medica Scandinavica*, **198**, 463–9.

26. Markiewicz, W., Houston, N. and DeBusk, R.F. (1977) Exercise testing soon after myocardial infarction. *Circulation*, **56**, 26–31.

27. De Busk, R.F. and Dennis, C.A. (1985) Submaximal pre-discharge exercise testing after acute myocardial infarction. Who needs it? *American Journal of Cardiology*, **55**, 499–500.

28. Kornbluch, I.H. and Michels, E. (1957) Outline of an exercise program for patients with myocardial infarction, *Pennsylvania Medical Journal*, **Dec**, 1575–8.

29. Cain, H.D., Frasher, W.G. and Stivelman, R. (1961) Graded activity program for safe return to self-care after myocardial infarction, *Journal of the American Medical Association*, **177**, 111–5.

30. Torkelson, L.O. (1964) Rehabilitation of the patient with acute myocardial infarction, *Journal of Chronic Diseases*, **17**, 685–704.
31. Chapman, C.B. and Fraser, R.S. (1954) Studies on the effect of exercise on cardiovascular function. III Cardiovascular response to exercise in patients with healed myocardial infarction, *Circulation*, **9**, 347–51.
32. Morris, J., Heady, J., Raffle, P., Roberts, C. and Parks, J. (1953) Coronary heart disease and physical activity of work, *Lancet*, **2**, 1053.
33. Fox, S.M. and Skinner, J.S. (1964) Physical activity and cardiovascular health, *American Journal of Cardiology*, **14**, 731–46.
34. Eckstein, R.W. (1957) Effect of exercise and coronary artery narrowing on coronary collateral circulation, *Circulation Research*, **5**, 230.
35. Gottheiner, V. (1986) Long-range strenuous sports training for cardiac reconditioning and rehabilitation, *American Journal of Cardiology*, **22**, 426–35.
36. Kellerman, J.J., Levy, M., Feldman, S. and Kariv, I. (1967) Rehabilitation of coronary patients, *Journal of Chronic Diseases*, **20**, 815–21.
37. Brunner, D. (1968) Active exercise for coronary patients, *Rehabilitation Record*, **Sept-Oct**, 29–31.
38. Zohman, L.R. and Tobis, J.S. (1967) The effect of exercise training on patients with angina pectoris, *Archives of Physical Medicine and Rehabilitation*, **48**, 525–32.
39. Hellerstein, H.K. and Ford, A.B. (1957) Rehabilitation of the cardiac patient, *Journal of the American Medical Association*, **164**, 225–31.
40. Hellerstein, H.K., Hirsch, E.Z., Cumler, W., Allen, L., Polster, S. and Zucker, N. (1963) Reconditioning of the coronary patient. Preliminary report. In W. Likoff and J.H. Moyer (eds), *Coronary Heart Disease*, New York: Grune and Stratton Inc.
41. Hellerstein, H.K. and Hornsten, T.R. (1966) Assessing and preparing the patient for return to a meaningful and productive life, *Journal of Rehabilitation*, **32**, 48–52.
42. Hellerstein, H.K., Hornsten, T.R., Goldbarg, A., Burlando, A.G., Friedman, E.H., Hirsch, E.Z. and Marik, S. (1967) The influence of active conditioning upon subjects with coronary artery disease: cardiorespiratory changes during training in 67 patients, *Canadian Medical Association Journal*, **96**, 758–9.
43. Hellerstein, H.K. (1968) Exercise therapy in coronary disease, *Bulletin of the New York Academy of Medicine*, **44**, 1028–47.
44. Barry, A.J., Daly, J.W., Pruett, E.D.R., Steinmetz, J.R., Birkhead, N.C. and Rodahl, K. (1966) Effects of physical training in patients who have had myocardial infarction, *American Journal of Cardiology*, **17**, 1–8.
45. Naughton, J. and McCoy, J.F. (1966) Observations on the relationship of physical activity to the serum cholesterol concentration of healthy men and cardiac patients, *Journal of Chronic Diseases*, **9**, 727–33.
46. Naughton, J., Bruhn, J. and Lategola, M. (1969) Rehabilitation following myocardial infarction, *American Journal of Medicine*, **46**, 725–34.

47. Rechnitzer, P.A., Yuhasz, M.S., Paivio, A., Pickard, H.A. and Lefcoe, N. (1967) Effects of a 24-week exercise programme on normal adults and patients with previous myocardial infarction, *British Medical Journal*, 1 734–5.

48. McPherson, B.D., Paivio, A., Yuhasz, M.S., Rechnitzer, P.A., Pickard, H.A. and Lefcoe, N.B. (1967) Psychological effects of an exercise program for post-infarct and normal adult men, *Journal of Sports Medicine*, 7, 95–102.

49. Varnauskas, E., Bergman, H., Hovk, P. and Bjorntorp, P. (1966) Haemodynamic effects of physical training in coronary patients, *Lancet*, 2, 8–12.

50. Frick, M.H. and Katila, M. (1968) Hemodynamic consequences of physical training after myocardial infarction, *Circulation*, **37**, 192–202.

51. Katila, M. and Frick, M.H. (1970) A two-year circulatory follow-up of physical training after myocardial infarction, *Acta Medica Scandinavica*, **187**, 95–100.

52. Clausen, J.P., Larsen, O.A. and Trap-Jensen, D. (1969) Physical training in the management of coronary artery disease, *Circulation*, **40**, 143–54.

Chapter 2

Cardiac Rehabilitation: Programme Structure, Content, Management and Administration

Summary

This chapter describes a structure which may be considered when providing a cardiac rehabilitation service. The content of the different phases of the rehabilitation process are discussed. Suggestions for staffing and administrative issues are made.

Introduction

When setting up a cardiac rehabilitation programme it is helpful to consider a structure which will cater for the needs of patients at the different stages of their disease and recovery process. Planning such a structure helps to clarify certain issues – e.g. what should be done, when, where, to whom and by whom. A logical way to divide these stages is to consider four phases, commencing with the in-patient stay, then the immediate post-discharge period, an intermediate post-discharge period and long-term maintenance. This is based on an assumption of hospital admission, but it may easily be adapted to cater for non-hospital admissions. The duration of each phase may vary, as may their content and the needs of the individual patient according to the availability of local resources (see Appendix 1).

The range of conditions which are considered eligible for cardiac rehabilitation will be dealt with in detail in the medical chapter and therefore will not be examined in depth here. However, it is important to mention that there are some people – e.g. women, ethnic minorities, the elderly, angina sufferers, and those with more serious cardiac disease (see Chapter 3) – who have special needs which are not always catered for. Little information has been available until recently about the management of women on CR programmes. It is now clear that women are less likely to partake of CR services than men[1].This is so for a variety of reasons, such as the age difference in the typical male and typical female cardiac patient (women typically, being up to 10 years older than men at the time of a first MI)[2]. It is also evident from research from the USA that women are more likely to have a range of other disorders, such as arthritis, which deter participation in CR programmes; they are also more likely to have transport difficulties, and their reports of encouragement from their physicians for CR programmes are rated as being less enthusiastic than the reports of their male counterparts[3]. Information on the experience of women, and on other important sub-groups such as older or disabled individuals, those from different cultural backgrounds and those living in areas remote from any organized programme, is urgently needed in the UK context if cardiac rehabilitation is to achieve the potential it offers in managing patient problems. Assessments of variations on the traditional hospital-based CR programmes may help in the coming decade to identify a range of service approaches that will best suit the diverse range of patients and situations in which a CR approach may be of benefit. One relatively neglected group to date has been children and adolescents with cardiac problems. Cardiac rehabilitation services could provide a major contribution to their development and to the successful management of their disease. Some evidence is available on the physical effects of exercise training[4] but the psychosocial difficulties and the impact of a CR programme on these for young people has not yet been explored. Management of these various groups needs to be addressed systematically in research, audit and consumer assessments over the next few years.

It should be noted that if the basic premise that coronary heart disease (CHD) is a *chronic* disease process, is accepted, the system should be designed to allow patients to 'travel' between the phases as their individual needs dictate, according to the stability or instability of their disease. The phases described will now be explored in more detail with the aim of introducing ideas which may be adapted to local resources, rather than producing the definitive system for all circumstances.

Phase One: in-patient stay

Hospital admission

Patients may be admitted to a coronary care unit (CCU) or directly to a medical or surgical ward, depending on their diagnosis and the facilities available at the local hospital. When planning a programme, it is important to consider what group of patients one can feasibly cater for within a programme, and whether a 'menu-based' approach – i.e. different options for different conditions – should be offered. It is more practicable to start small, and then expand to cater for a wider range of conditions in the future, when staff have gained the confidence and expertise to do so.

The issues to consider for in-patient needs include:

■ Reassurance
■ Information

- Risk factor assessment
- Risk stratification
- Education
- Mobilization
- Discharge planning
- Involvement and support of partner/family.

Reassurance

The provision of reassurance should cover not only the immediate medical issues but also vocational and financial matters, as these are often foremost in the patient's mind at this stage. Access to an occupational therapist and/or social worker in addition to nursing and medical staff, may go far to alleviate the patient's anxiety in these matters. Many cardiac rehabilitation programmes do not start 'active' rehabilitation until some weeks after discharge[5]. Even if this is so, it is helpful to encourage a positive attitude to recovery from the first day of admission onwards, so that patients can be reassured that having a cardiac event does not signify a completely negative future outlook. Rehabilitation should in fact commence from the initial identification of the CHD patient.

It is most important at this point to attempt to establish what misconceptions the patient may have about CHD[6], and to deal with these in a realistic manner, as this will strongly influence the patient's attitude towards potential recovery (see Chapter 6). If specialist rehabilitation staff are available, they may carry out ward visits. These may be arranged on a one-to-one basis, as a group session, or both. If the resources are not available to provide this, then the existing ward staff may be used to provide this part of the service, but it is important to ensure that the information given is consistent and of a high standard. A recent report from the Audit Commission[7] highlights a number of issues concerning communication between hospitals and patients. Some of the problems identified include professionals not talking to each other, and therefore failing to co-ordinate patient care. Furthermore, the report notes that inadequate, inconsistent and contradictory information is often given in a hurry without time for questions. Guidelines regarding rehabilitation advice and mobilization as an in-patient should be negotiated, agreed and available for *all* staff involved with cardiac patients. It is useful to establish an agreement between the medical staff whose patients may be referred, and the staff involved in providing information, to ensure that the patient does not suffer from perceiving a conflict between the professionals involved, otherwise their confidence in the overall service may be reduced and their adherence to medical recommendations lowered.

The practice of using ex-patients to visit new patients in hospital or at home may be considered but should be treated with caution. It is essential that a careful screening of the volunteers is carried out if such a resource is to be utilized. Patients may be extremely vulnerable in the early stages of their recovery, and an inappropriate visit, even if well-intentioned, could do more harm than good.

If considering using volunteers, questions to ask are:

- What is the motivation of this volunteer?
- Can he or she
  - communicate well?
  - listen as well as give information?
  - be provided with some training and guidelines?
  - keep to the guidelines provided ?
- Is there any way to monitor the volunteer's progress and evaluate the service, so that its impact can be established?

It is also important not to impose this service on the patient simply because it may be available and inexpensive. Permission from the patient should always be sought before arranging such a visit, whether to an in-patient or after discharge.

Information/education

Advice needs to be provided in both a written and verbal form; neither alone is sufficient. Written information should be assessed for simplicity and clarity and attractive presentation. Many Trust hospitals now have a mechanism for vetting the literature produced for patient use by individual departments such as an Ethics Committee or a Literature Work Group. This is considered part of the 'corporate image', as the quality of printed information reflects the image of the hospital. It is wise, therefore, to ascertain local protocols and standards for presentation before producing new information packages. If information is to be translated into other languages, it is wise to check with the interpreter that although cultural differences must be taken into account, the essential meaning of the information is not radically changed during the process of translation. Verbal information needs to be pitched at the level appropriate to that individual and his or her partner or family. The assumption that everyone is literate is an inappropriate one to make, and not everyone is prepared to admit that he or she cannot read. Staff should be alert to the fact that the patient who does not appear to be taking in written information may in fact be unable to comprehend it. Videos may be used, especially during admission, and they may be useful to stimulate discussion, but they should not be seen as an adequate substitute for individual counselling.

Risk factor assessment

Assessment will include both an overall assessment of the individual needs and more specifically an assessment of the coronary risk factors involved. Information collected will include traditional demographic details but may vary tremendously in type of data recorded and methods of collection and storage. It may also involve more than one discipline to achieve an overall assessment.

Information collected may include:

- Family history of CHD
- Personal history of CHD
- Other relevant medical history
- Smoking history
- Dietary habits and cholesterol profile
- Body mass index (height and weight) or waist to hip ratio
- Blood pressure and history of hypertension
- Diabetes
- Physical activity levels: activities of daily living and general functional capacity
- Emotional status
- Individual behavioural style, e.g. type A behaviour pattern; hostility
- Prognostic evaluation
- Risk stratification
- Socioeconomic status
- Vocational status, and any licensing implications, e.g. driving
- Leisure activities.

It may not be possible to collect all the relevant information during admission as some data may not be available until after further investigations, e.g. graded exercise testing. However, a user-friendly data collection system will be invaluable in terms of clinical audit and programme evaluation and the importance of this should not be underestimated at this stage. The process of audit and evaluation will be discussed later in this chapter.

Mobilization

Mobilization needs to address two issues: prevention of complications, e.g. deep venous thrombosis and pulmonary embolus, and increasing the patient's confidence in preparation for discharge by activities appropriate to the home environment, such as climbing stairs, showering or bathing. This is another issue where agreement between all the professionals concerned must be reached if the patient is to feel confident about coping at home with activities of daily living. This is also where careful assessment of individual needs is vital and where questions such as whether patients live alone or with support, or whether they are themselves caring for another person all need to be addressed. These questions are closely related to discharge planning and the Community Care Act. It may be necessary to involve other members of the team – e.g. the occupational therapist to carry out a home assessment; evaluation by the social worker or possibly referral for assessment after discharge by a member of the primary healthcare team.

Mobilization in hospital is often via a standard format which increases rigidly from the first day through to discharge. It is more flexible to perceive the patient going through *stages* of mobilization rather than *days*. It may be helpful to have a structure to work from, and this can be based on the severity of the cardiac event[8]. Each individual should be allowed to progress at a pace suitable to him/her rather than be fitted into a format which suits only the standard care plan, thus not taking important clinical (e.g. infarct size) or patient (e.g. age or confidence) factors into account. Patients who may be disabled and wheelchair-bound should have a careful assessment made of their particular needs. There should be no reason to exclude them from any of the Phase Two activities, and they may benefit from an exercise programme tailored to their individual capabilities.

Discharge planning

All in-patients should have a discharge plan commencing from the time of admission. This could be used by the ward staff to refer the patient to the rehabilitation team. A care plan may have been written by the ward staff, liaising with the rehabilitation staff . The rehabilitation team may have their own care plan, having discussed with the patient, current lifestyle and options for change. A careful assessment will need to be made regarding those patients who may have a previous history of significant psychiatric disorder. Staff will need to assess in this instance whether there is a risk of the group dynamics of a CR programme being disrupted, to the detriment of other patients' recovery. If this seems possible or likely, then staff will need to consider what other options may be available, to ensure they cater for the individual's needs without putting the group under additional pressure, and without draining the staff resources unduly.

Another group of patients who may require careful thought as to their eligibility to participate are those where the diagnosis is uncertain, or identified as non-cardiac chest pain. There is an inherent danger in labelling people with a cardiac diagnosis if it is not absolutely confirmed, as once that seed is planted it can be very difficult to eradicate and their lives can be dramatically affected for no good reason[9]. In those where cardiac disease has, as far as possible, been ruled out (i.e. by normal angiographic results) it may be hard to enable them to lead a normal life again. Although the principle that they would gain confidence from an exercise programme may apply, entering them into a cardiac rehabilitation programme is not necessarily appropriate as it reinforces the 'cardiac' labelling. An alternative might be referral to a GP exercise prescription programme, if one is available locally.

Good practice may include, for example:

- A maximum time period within which all in-patients are to be visited;
- An assessment tool to be commenced within the same time period;
- A discharge/care plan for each individual including follow-up appointments.

Ideally, all notes kept on the patient should be multidisciplinary, as should the care plan[10]. As this may be difficult to implement, the key to a successful plan is simplicity: an ambitious revamping of the patient's entire lifestyle is less likely to work than a plan capitalizing on patient motivation to make a few simple changes. If patients can achieve *one* change successfully (e.g. give up smoking), then they are more likely to be inclined to try other changes, but these need to be introduced gradually over a period of time and in some order of priority, so that they are not overloaded. It is important not to be judgemental when advising on lifestyle change, as this tends to be counterproductive!

In some areas, the idea of patient-held records and a greater degree of 'shared care' between hospital and community staff is being explored and developed. This is particularly relevant in areas where patients may have to travel between one hospital and another for investigations and treatment. Even if travel is not involved, anything which facilitates improved communication between members of the hospital staff, the primary healthcare team, the rehabilitation staff and the patient must be seen as a step forward. It may also encourage patients to take some responsibility for their own health status, by being increasingly involved in decisions about lifestyle change and treatment.

The 'ripple' effect of health education for patients promoting primary prevention among the rest of the family is another issue not to be underestimated. Much useful work can be done when discussing lifestyle change with the patient to encourage other family members to make the same changes. Not only will this help the patient's motivation and compliance, but it will hopefully reduce the potential of disease in other family members. In instances where, for example, hypercholesterolaemia is discovered, liaison with the primary healthcare team for family screening will be essential for long-term follow-up.

Partner/family involvement

Ideally, the patient's partner and family will be given the opportunity to become involved in the process of discussion and discharge planning at an early stage. The amount of reassurance needed by partners should not be underestimated, even though they may appear to be coping well. Studies have shown that the partners of those with heart disease often lie awake at night just so that they can hear their partner breathing and be reassured that they are still alive[11]. The pattern of over-protection will be familiar to many, where the 'sick' partner is restricted at home, functioning well below the level of activity s/he could reasonably be expected to do, and this situation may well lead to unnecessary conflict. Advice on what level of activity is suitable and general reassurance to those at home will be invaluable in tackling these issues – as will telephone access if possible (See also Chapters 5 and 6).

The issue of teaching resuscitation techniques on CR programmes is one which causes some division of opinion. Some feel that it is a positive approach for those who have a partner or family member with heart disease and who may wish to feel reassured by knowing that they have the basic skills to act in an emergency. Others feel that it reinforces the negative aspects of anxiety by implying that an emergency is likely to happen and that there is an expectation that they should be able to cope. It is certainly a subject which should be introduced in a manner which allows complete freedom of choice to those concerned and puts no pressure on them to participate if they do not want to. The timing of the introduction of such an issue needs to be carefully considered as well.

If programme co-ordinators do wish to provide training, several options are available. The St John Ambulance Brigade run training courses in most areas, geared towards the fact that if every member of the public can do something in any emergency situation, this may help to save a life. Presenting resuscitation in this way takes the pressure off the implied responsibility of specifically coping with the management of a member of one's own family. Alternatively, partners or family may feel more comfortable having a member of the rehabilitation team or other hospital staff training them in some basic resuscitation techniques.

The 'Heart Manual'

The 'Heart Manual' is a six-week home-based post-MI rehabilitation programme, designed by a CR team and supported by the British Heart Foundation and the Scottish Office. It was evaluated through a controlled trial in a district general hospital[6], and further evaluation is continuing. It is currently in use in more than 80 hospitals and in the last three years over 5000 patients have used it.

The patient begins the programme on discharge, following an initial structured interview with the Heart Manual facilitator. This is usually a nurse, but it could be any health worker who has completed the two-day training programme. Before discharge, the patient and his or her partner are introduced to the working materials. These consist of a workbook in six parts and two cassette tapes. Following discharge, the patient's compliance is checked and motivation boosted by a series of contacts with the facilitator. This may either be through brief telephone calls, or through home or hospital visits. At the end of the six week period, the patient is reassessed using a structured interview and questionnaires. Six weeks has been shown to be the ideal time to identify those who are going to have a poor rehabilitation outcome, and those patients demonstrating problems at this assessment can then enter a more intensive CR programme, or receive individual attention from the relevant healthcare professional.

A particularly interesting development, pioneered in Dumfries and Galloway, in Scotland, has been the adoption of the Heart Manual across whole health districts. For example, one health authority provides it to all post-MI patients and each GP practice has two trained facilitators who can then provide further contact for patients and their partners. In this way, all post-MI patients, including those who are not admitted to hospital (except for a small number who are too ill) receive a basic CR package, then have their ongoing needs assessed. This may provide a model for provision of CR, particularly in rural areas, or any area where transport and/or access to a more traditional hospital-based CR programme is difficult.

Bearing in mind the numbers of patients eligible for CR, it may also provide a useful screening process by meeting the needs of 'uncomplicated' patients, thereby freeing resources to be used for more difficult groups or individuals. However, it should be stressed that the Heart Manual should be regarded as only one part of a CR service and not as a cheap alternative to a comprehensive service that can meet the needs of all cardiac patients. (For further information see Useful Addresses.)

Phase Two: immediate post-discharge (4–6 weeks)

Phase Two is a phase which is currently neglected in many cardiac rehabilitation programmes but which is nevertheless a crucial time period for patients in terms of adjustment to change. It can be a time in which cardiac rehabilitation professionals capitalize on the patient's motivation to change.

It is also a stage which logically focuses on health education and the resumption of physical activity. This may apply to post-myocardial infarction patients during the initial phase of healing of the myocardium, or post-coronary artery bypass graft (CABG) patients during the initial postoperative healing phase. For others who do not have a healing period to go through, such as those with angina, it may simply be their first opportunity to have access to a health education programme relevant to their disease. This is a point at which direct general practitioner referrals may be introduced to the programme.

It may also be seen as a useful two-way process: offering an education programme over a period of weeks enables the patients to absorb information in manageable chunks; it also enables the professionals involved to assess their progress on a regular basis and to identify problems at an early stage. For those in whom denial is present, perhaps as an early coping mechanism, Phase Two also ensures that contact is maintained during this stage, possibly helping the patient to go through the process of acceptance; if this process does not appear to be taking place, then it helps to identify those who may need further help in adjusting to their disease. Problems can then be referred for management to an appropriate agent, i.e. the hospital team or the GP. The importance of this process, sometimes known as 'surveillance', should not be underestimated in the early detection of complications and the potential to reduce unnecessary re-admissions.

There are several ways to consider follow-up of patients up during Phase Two:

- Staff make follow-up telephone calls;
- Patients have access to a telephone service which they can use as required, or at specific times;
- Staff make home visits;
- Patients attend individual appointments;
- Patients attend group sessions.

There are advantages and disadvantages for each of these options and these are discussed below.

Follow-up

Telephone follow-up

Advantages: Telephone follow-up will be less time-consuming than home visits and less costly. It can provide reassurance and an answering machine service can be useful in allowing freedom of contact for the patient and family. Staff can use a checklist to ensure that important follow-up points are not omitted.

Disadvantages: Staff need to possess excellent communication skills in order to detect verbal clues as they are denied benefit of visual contact and clues from body language. Staff also need skill in drawing out information: not everyone is comfortable on the end of a telephone, particularly when dealing with emotional issues. If there are not the cardiac rehabilitation resources to provide this service, is the CCU or are the ward staff equipped to do so in terms of skills and time? There is also a risk of patient dependency, and it can be difficult trying to prevent people from using this kind of service inappropriately. Answering machines can be inhibiting and de-humanizing to some people. Telephones with 24-hour staff coverage, such as in a coronary care unit, may be more friendly, but the staff may not always have the time to talk. In lower socioeconomic groups (who may have a higher incidence of heart disease) there may not be easy access to a telephone – in which case, this form of routine follow-up is impossible.

Home visits

Advantages: Patients may feel more comfortable at home, away from the hospital environment; thus home visits may allow for a fuller patient assessment. It may be easier also to involve the partner and family, and to assess how they interact together. If the patient has been a GP referral rather than a hospital admission, a home visit may be the first opportunity to assess whether the patient is, in fact, an appropriate referral. If called out for a specific reason, the problem will be easier to identify and resolve than to attempt to visualize on the end of a telephone. There may be an increased empathy in this setting as staff are removed from many of the distracting or distancing aspects of hospital care. Home visits may help also to keep channels open during, for example, the post-CABG euphoria stage when patients may not always realize at the time how much support they do need. The time involved will usually be $\frac{1}{2}$–1 hour, excluding travel.

Disadvantages: Home visits can be time-consuming and therefore expensive – both in the cost of the time and in the actual mileage allowance, when allowing for travel between base and client. It is also easy to get side-tracked away from clinical issues, and parameters need to be set. Staff may feel vulnerable on their own in an unknown setting, and during travel; staff safety should not be ignored. Other professionals may also be doing home visits and the consistency of information may be at risk unless this has been established with all those concerned. Professional rivalry may exist. One professional may visit and do a blood pressure check and when another professional visits, the patient's expectations of this being repeated are then raised. Staff need experience to recognize conflict in the home and may be in danger of becoming 'pig-in-the-middle' between the patient and the partner/family. Home visiting may also encourage sick role beliefs and behaviour – i.e. patients believe they are not well enough to go out and so have to be visited at home (although this can be minimized by specific advice on the expected level of activity from experienced staff).

Individual counselling sessions

Advantages: Individual counselling sessions may allow for more privacy than a group session and also allow the individual the freedom to discuss any queries or concerns alone or as a couple or family. All patients require differing degrees of support which can be offered by all members of the multidisciplinary team, but if structured, in-depth counselling is required, then patients need to be referred to a professional with an appropriate qualification in counselling or therapy, or to a team member receiving competent supervision (see Chapter 6).

Disadvantages: Sessions are time-consuming and therefore costly. In the short term, they also do not allow for any peer group support or interaction. Staff may also encounter problems of dependency (as can occur in counselling) and so need to be equipped with the skills to deal with this situation should it arise. Furthermore, staff need to be able to recognize their own limitations in counselling and to know when to refer the patient to a more experienced professional.

Group sessions

Advantages: Group, as opposed to individual, counselling sessions allow for peer group as well as professional support; patients may gain much from meeting others with similar conditions/problems. Group sessions allow patients to listen to answers to queries which others may ask, which they themselves may have felt too inhibited to raise. These sessions are time-effective for staff and, depending on the timing and the structure of the session, may allow for some individual counselling as well, where appropriate.

Disadvantages: Some patients may not enjoy a group atmosphere and may feel intimidated about asking questions in front of others. Others may dominate the group and personalize every issue. The range of individuals will vary considerably and it may be hard to form a cohesive group, which interacts well together. The size of the group may affect the quality of the discussion. The beneficial effects of the group sessions may only last while members are attending the group and may dissipate as soon as the group 'disbands'.

Education sessions

Many factors affect the individual's capacity to learn. Life experience will have shaped each person's perceptions and expectations of his or her current situation.

Many teaching sessions are oriented towards giving information on a variety of topics rather than exploring theories of adult learning. Unless the 'teacher' spends some time assessing the different needs of the group members, it will be difficult to target sessions at the right level.

Girdano and Dusek[12] in their work on changing health behaviour have examined what makes an individual ready to learn, and have defined

> ... readiness as the possession of behaviours, attitudes, skills, and concomitant resources that make it possible for individuals to incorporate a new health behaviour into a permanent lifestyle.

This hypothesis would imply that it is more profitable to spend some time exploring attitudes prior to imparting information. The ten steps which they have identified in the scale of readiness to learn are as follows. The individual:

- Understands the concepts;
- Values the change, verbalizes as good or right;
- Believes new behaviour is possible;
- Visualizes a new behaviour with low ambiguity;
- Believes in ability to change behaviour;
- Can see proof of attainment;
- Possesses new skills;
- Practises new skills on regular basis;
- Practises skills in real-life situation;
- Adopts new behaviour as lifestyle – without thinking about it.

Helping people to learn may be seen as helping them to move up this scale, as opposed to feeding them with information – however comprehensive the information package may seem. Adults' motivation to learn also tends to be affected by factors which are immediately relevant to their lives[13], rather than concepts which they may not relate to themselves. This again emphasizes the need to assess the individual's perceptions and expectations in order to satisfy learning needs . It can sometimes be difficult for healthcare professionals to accept that people may not want to learn or to change, even though by not changing they are perceived to be putting their health at risk. One of the objectives of the CR personnel should be the achievement of change through choice, rather than by imposition. The timing of education is important, and the earlier it can be incorporated, the better. Otherwise, patients feel that the immediate relevance is lost, and may justifiably ask why they have not been given important information sooner.

Feedback

Questionnaires may or may not be the best way to evaluate patient information: they may provide an insight but sometimes only supply superficial information.

Much depends on the design of the questionnaire: whether it addresses the questions which the patients feel are the most relevant[10], whether it is easy to use and, of course, whether the patient is literate. Listening to the type of questions asked during a group session may be a better way of assessing the level of understanding of patients.

Teaching aids

The use of audiovisual aids, handouts and other material needs to be examined for their suitability, readability, clarity of expression and length. Programmes will need to cater for a wide range of ages, mental abilities and cultural backgrounds and will need a range of resources accordingly. Studies have shown that some of the standard literature used as handouts can score as difficult on readability tests[14] and, as mentioned earlier in this chapter, translated material may not always have the same impact as the original intended, due to changes during translation. Videos may be a useful alternative and can be used to provoke a discussion; however, they can quickly appear dated. If used frequently, they can also become stale to the staff using them and it may become more difficult to present them with enthusiasm.

'Personalized' material

Can the material be tailored to the individual in any way? The patient may be more inclined to take in and use information if there are parts that can be filled in, relating to their own condition and bringing the subject to a personal level.

Practical issues

Practicalities – for example organizing the classroom to accommodate the hard-of-hearing and visually impaired – need to be planned for. Temperature, adequate ventilation and general comfort are also going to influence the success of teaching sessions.

Topics to be covered may include:

- The disease process
- Investigations
- Treatment
- Risk factors: smoking
  diet
  blood pressure
  physical activity
  cholesterol levels
- Medication
- Stress management and relaxation techniques

- Physical activity: activities of daily living
  sexual relationships
  exercise
- Driving
- Insurance
- Return to work
- Resuscitation
- Social and leisure activities.

Attendance

Issues to consider with regard to educational programme attendance include the following:

- How will patients take part in these sessions: by invitation or expectation?
- Can the partner/family attend if they so wish?
- Should the sessions be presented as a routine part of follow-up or will patients be given the option to attend only if they wish to do so?

The implications of the latter system, in view of early denial, are that some people will not take up the offer of these sessions because they do not perceive that they have a problem or a need for information.

Phase Three: Intermediate post-discharge

Phase Three is sometimes regarded purely as 'the exercise phase'. This is a misconception, as the importance of psychosocial interventions should not be regarded as any less than that of exercise-oriented interventions (see Chapter 6). Also, if it has not been possible to incorporate a Phase Two stage into the programme, then this may be the period in which not only exercise, but also education and lifestyle change factors need to be included.

Issues of exercise prescription are examined in Chapter 4 and so will not be dealt with in depth here. One of the issues of paramount importance in setting-up an exercise programme is that of patient safety. This is influenced by several factors. These are:

- Risk stratification and the identification of the high risk patient;
- Inclusion/exclusion criteria for exercise sessions;
- Experience of staff;
- Resuscitation resources;
- Health and safety issues regarding premises and equipment.

Safety in a cardiac rehabilitation programme results from careful planning and adherence to standards within the programme[15]. It cannot be emphasized strongly enough that medical screening and assessment, risk stratification, exercise prescription, supervision and monitoring are key elements of programme safety and should not be ignored for the sake of expediency.

Vocational support

Patients may need referral for occupational therapy for help in returning to work. This may have already taken place if a problem was identified at an earlier stage. An analysis of the patient's working environment – in respect of it's physical and psychological demands – and an assessment of his/her ability to return to work may be carried out by the occupational therapist. For example, the level of physical activity required to perform certain tasks may need to be assessed and targeted with graded activity programmes and individual vocational-related exercise prescription. Other factors that may need examination include time management, assertion skills and problem-solving techniques.

Staff may need to liaise with a patient's employer or occupational health nurse to:

- Report on the patient's progress;
- Emphasize the need for a change in the pattern of a patient's employment;
- Suggest a graded return to work.

Should a patient *not* be able to return to previous employment, referral to a disablement employment advisor or vocational advisor at a local job centre may be appropriate. However, for every patient, whether in employment or not, it is just as important to consider return to all activities of daily living, i.e. vocational, social and leisure, in order to maintain self-esteem. If confidence in ability is lacking in any of these areas, a graded activity programme may be appropriate.

From the start of Phase Three, it is important to be planning for the transition into Phase Four and long-term maintenance of changes. It is not helpful for the individual to be closely supervised for a number of weeks, only to be moved into Phase Four without adequate preparation. Some people may exhibit strong dependent behaviour and it is important that a CR programme does not promote this. An inexperienced professional may inadvertently, through dedication and enthusiasm, create dependency. This may initially enhance work satisfaction and sense of purpose, but in the longer term, it is unhelpful to both staff and patient. A classic situation occurs where patients are highly motivated to exercise and maintain changes while they feel looked after on a CR programme, but once the formal programme is complete, the motivation rapidly dissipates.

Individual goals should be discussed with each CR participant and the approach should be one of facilitating the achievement of these goals and fostering independence at an early stage. It is also important to encourage this independence from the point of proving to individual participants that they are capable of managing on their own; that the reality of everyday life is that they are not going to be permanently monitored!

It is helpful to set criteria (both physical and psychological) for moving from one phase to another, as not everyone will progress on the same time scale. If the time scale is altered due to a change in the patient's condition, then this must be explained to the patient, otherwise it may cause great anxiety.

Three criteria to achieve for advancement from Phase Three to Phase Four, have been specified as goals by the Massachusetts Association for Cardiovascular and Pulmonary Rehabilitation[16]. They aim to promote:

- Significant improvement in functional capacity;
- Psychological adaptation to chronic disease;
- The foundation of behavioural and lifestyle changes required for continued risk factor modification.

More specific objectives may be related to the level of risk stratification and may include the patient:

- Demonstrating an ability to exercise safely and effectively, according to an individual exercise prescription;
- Being able to monitor own heart rate or use scale of perceived exertion effectively;
- Being able to recognize warning signs and symptoms and take appropriate action (e.g. stop/reduce exercise level, take GTN);
- Being able to identify specific goals for long-term maintenance of lifestyle change and risk factor reduction, relating to own personal history;
- Being able to identify goals relating to psychosocial interventions, and plan necessary support needed.

The time scale recommended to achieve these goals is attendance at 36 sessions over a three to six-month period, although it should be noted that this is one set of specific recommendations, and the principle of a flexible, individually oriented time frame should be applied in general.

Phase Four: Long-term maintenance

Phase Four constitutes two main components:

1. Long-term maintenance of individual goals;
2. Professional monitoring of clinical status and follow-up of general progress.

This will involve close liaison with the primary healthcare team for follow-up of clinical issues such as:

- Raised cholesterol levels;
- Hypertension;
- Stability of angina;
- Medication review (including effectiveness and compliance).

and for risk factor reduction, lifestyle changes and general coping mechanisms, in such areas as:

- Smoking;
- Weight control;
- Physical activity, including activities of daily living;
- Psychosocial adjustment;
- Vocational support.

It is helpful for the primary healthcare team to receive a letter from the CR programme at the end of Phase Three. This should detail the patient's progress, the goals achieved, and those which have not yet been achieved. Details of any follow-up planned by the CR team will also help the GP to plan involvement in the process of long-term monitoring of risk factor reduction. This kind of information sharing is an essential link in the chain of communication. It is important when sending such letters to a surgery, to request that they will be circulated to the team and not just to the GP, otherwise they may not reach all the relevant team members.

It may be possible to enable patients to continue to exercise using the facilities they are already familiar with at the CR programme site; this may encourage compliance as people often prefer familiar surroundings and may have peer support to maintain their motivation[17]. It can also be used as an opportunity to generate income, as there is not an ethical problem in charging a small fee for long-term use of exercise facilities, once participants have graduated from the immediate care and follow-up phases. Otherwise, CR co-ordinators may wish to advise patients of alternative exercise facilities available locally and a local sports centre may be willing to offer patients a reduced fee at off-peak times. This may also help to encourage groups or 'buddies' exercising together, which in turn may maintain motivation levels.

The concept of exercise and health promotion going hand-in-hand is not a new one and in some areas, where GP exercise prescription schemes are being run at sports and leisure facilities, there may be a readiness to form a cooperative venture in utilizing particular times for access to the facilities. Over recent years, many GP practices have teamed up with their local leisure centre to provide a health-related exercise referral service. The aim of such schemes is generally to provide a safe introduction to exercise for sedentary individuals whose health may benefit from increased levels of appropriate physical activity. Schemes are mainly designed to cater for patients who have one or more low-level CHD risk factors, e.g. moderately raised blood pressure or cholesterol, a body mass index of between

26–30, those suffering from anxiety or stress, or those with a famil
CHD. Other criteria may include impaired strength or mobility. Sch
generally accept patients at high risk of CHD or those with establi
Schemes are mainly managed on a day-to-day basis by exercise
without the presence of medical personnel or support from other qualified
professionals and therefore are not appropriate for recent CHD patients or for
those who have not previously undergone supervised exercise rehabilitation. GP
exercise schemes may, however, provide a suitable stepping-stone in the transition
from supervised CR to exercising independently, and may be appropriate for CR
'graduates'. It should be stressed that this level of supervision is not suitable as –
and should in no way be perceived as such – a cheaper alternative to Phase Three
care.

Alternatively, individuals may prefer to exercise independently and part of their
criteria of progression from Phase Three to Phase Four may involve helping them
to set a safe and realistic maintenance programme, and a means of reviewing this
as necessary.

Cardiac support groups

There may already be a local Cardiac Support Group, this could be functioning
independently or could be one in which the CR team is involved. The British
Heart Foundation (BHF) has set up a network for such groups to provide
national support. This offers several advantages, including:

- Insurance cover;
- Two free tickets for members of the group, to attend relevant conferences;
- Support and advice from regional advisors;
- Newsletters and bulletins;
- Access to up-to-date publications;
- Networking with other groups.

Such groups, whether BHF-affiliated or not, may be particularly helpful to
partners and family in providing an opportunity to discuss feelings with others in
a similar situation. If there is not such a group locally, the BHF provide a useful
information package on how to set one up. This may help to avoid some of the
potential pitfalls which can arise. The BHF address can be found in the list of
addresses at the back of this publication.

Management and administration

Core functions

The core functions of a cardiac rehabilitation team may be perceived as:

- Individual patient assessment;

- Management and provision of service;
- Adequate emergency response.

If taken in conjunction with Phases One to Four detailed earlier, this provides a framework to plan and assess the feasibility of implementing a safe and effective programme.

Individual patient assessment

Clinical assessment is described in Chapter 3. Different members of the multi-disciplinary team will be involved in the processes covered earlier in this chapter, such as those relating to risk factor assessment, discharge care planning, setting realistic goals for lifestyle changes and long-term maintenance. Documentation relating to these processes is again varied. Each programme tends to develop its own format depending on local staffing and resources. Examples of forms currently in use may be obtained from the addresses given at the end of this chapter.

Management and provision of service

The fact that cardiac rehabilitation needs to be regarded as a multidisciplinary field has already been discussed. The staffing of programmes will depend largely on funding and local resources. As yet, there is little available in terms of specialist training in this field although it is an issue currently under review by a sub-committee of the British Association for Cardiac Rehabilitation. It is expected that a training system will be developed and that accreditation for training will be sought from a reputable academic institution in order to ensure that high standards are set and achieved. Healthcare professionals who might be part of a cardiac rehabilitation team (in alphabetical order) include:

- Cardiologists
- Dieticians
- Exercise physiologists
- General physicians, with an interest in cardiology
- General practitioners
- Occupational therapists
- Pharmacists
- Physiotherapists
- Psychologists
- Registered nurses
- Social workers.

Others who may be involved include those working in:

- Counselling;

- Health promotion;
- Look After Your Heart tutors;
- Primary healthcare teams;
- Sports/leisure;
- Stress management;
- Vocational advice.

It is impossible, however, to stipulate the particular combination of staff required. In the USA, staff roles and levels of competency are clearly defined, but in the UK we are not yet in a position to set such standards. The core funding arrangements differ greatly, and the lack of training available militates against setting prescriptive standards of qualifications and experience. It is therefore important, when planning or reviewing staffing, to examine the core competencies which are possessed as a team, to ensure that the best mix of staff abilities is available in the service which is offered.

Combined knowledge base

The combined skills/knowledge base should include:

- Anatomy and physiology of cardiac function;
- The process of cardiovascular disease;
- Health psychology;
- Theories of adult education;
- Theories of motivation and change;
- Counselling skills;
- Exercise physiology;
- Individual exercise prescription;
- Management of emergencies;
- Nutrition and weight loss;
- Vocational advice;
- Audit and evaluation;
- Research;
- Management and administration.

In order to provide a comprehensive service, qualifications additional to the core professional qualifications of the team members, e.g. teaching, counselling or exercise skills, may be desirable.

Co-ordination of service

The identification of a programme co-ordinator is an essential step in ensuring the efficient provision of service. Although a mixture of team members is needed, one person must have the overall responsibility for the day-to-day running of the service. In addition to any patient-oriented activities, this role may include:

- The formation, development and review of policies and procedures for the programme;
- Budget management, liaison with the business manager, contributing to the performance and business plans;
- Regular communication with team members and liaison with other departments and staff, such as the Medical Directorate;
- Staff training, development and performance review;
- Participation in data collection, audit and evaluation of the programme;
- Initiation of/collaboration in research related to the programme;
- Ordering and maintenance of equipment;
- Health and Safety responsibilities.

Provision must also take into account the facilities available to the CR programme, and the support of key local elements, such as the cardiologist(s) and the health authority. Without local approval and co-operation between the different bodies, it becomes very difficult to implement a programme successfully. Although programmes have been set up in areas where there is a lack of either general or specific support, this can lead to immense pressures on the staff members attempting to provide a service, with a potential for problems for staff themselves, the service, or both.

The British Cardiac Society Working Party report[18] highlights the fact that the lack of direct cardiologist involvement in CR significantly affects the development of local programmes. It is to be hoped that the growing interest and concern amongst CR professionals, and the increase in research-based evidence of the benefits and effectiveness of CR, will help to convince those who remain sceptical.

Facilities

The facilities currently available for CR throughout the UK vary from programmes with no dedicated facilities to units which are fully equipped with offices, gyms and teaching areas. They also vary between hospital and community-based programmes. Some of these programmes may be linked, having an initial phase in the hospital and progressing to a community-based phase at a later date. The space required is often underestimated, and may be difficult to negotiate in a climate where internal charges may be made for the use of hospital premises. The following points need to be considered in relation to facilities:

- **Office space**

Staff need to store records in a secure and confidential manner, i.e. in a lockable filing cabinet. A telephone is essential and an answer-machine provides a useful contact point for staff and patients. The telephone needs to be situated with some privacy so that confidentiality can be maintained. If a computer is available, this will make data storage and retrieval much easier.

■ **Counselling**

Privacy is essential for counselling purposes and a comfortable space which can be used without interruptions needs to be available.

■ **Education**

If running group sessions, there needs to be access to an area large enough to cater for the group comfortably. This means not only the size of the room, but the type of seating, temperature and ventilation, catering facilities for drinks, and toilet facilities. Ease of access to the area needs to be assessed for those with disabilities.

■ **Exercise**

The same considerations apply to exercise facilities. Temperature control and humidity are even more important. Humidity should be maintained at approximately 65% and temperature controlled at between 65–72°F. If, during seasonal variations, it is impossible to maintain these conditions, staff responsible should seriously consider closing down exercise sessions, so as not to put cardiac patients further at risk by exercising in extremes of heat or cold.

□ Drinking water should be available, to replace fluids lost during exercise.
□ Ideally, separate changing rooms and showers should be available.
□ Patients should be warned about theft of valuables, and have access to secure lockers if possible.
□ An area should be accessible equipped with chairs and a couch, and a telephone should be situated for easy access in case of an emergency.
□ A first aid kit should be present at every exercise session, and a suitably trained member of staff designated as a first-aider.

Health and safety issues

These include:

■ Fire regulations and access to exits;
■ Use and maintenance of electrical equipment, e.g. audio-visual aids;
■ Safe placement of exercise equipment;
■ Maintenance of exercise equipment;
■ Maintenance of resuscitation equipment.

Insurance

The CR programme co-ordinator must ensure that adequate insurance cover exists for whatever sessions are being run. Patients are normally covered by the general hospital insurance if sessions are held on site, but if sessions are held on other premises, such as a sports centre or community centre, then it is the responsibility of the CR programme to ensure that insurance and liability have been investigated. Support groups should also be aware of this, particularly if they are running any kind of exercise session, and advice can be obtained from the BHF on this issue.

Audit

There are many 'buzz words' in the healthcare system at the moment and it is easy to become immune to the importance of the issues at stake when they are used repetitively at every opportunity. However, the process of audit should be perceived as a useful tool for all CR programme co-ordinators in evaluating the standards and quality of the service they are providing.

The audit cycle, in its simplest form, is a process of setting standards, measuring and comparing practice with standards, identifying and implementing change, and then either continuously or intermittently reviewing the process. To be successful, audit should benefit everyone involved. The following useful summary is provided in the Department of Health Report: Clinical Audit in the Nursing and Therapy Professions[19]. The goals to be achieved in audit include:

- *Outcome of audit:* improvement in the quality of care, and best achievable outcomes;
- *Infrastructure:* clinical audit should be fully embedded in the National Health Service;
- *Education and training:* audit should be an integral part of all professional education;
- *National projects:* where results should have a wide application and be transferable;
- *Standards:* audit should include standard setting which can be measured against practice;
- *Purchasing:* audit findings should inform the contracting process.

The report also emphasizes that the trend is towards multiprofessional clinical audit, and that by involving the perspectives of many disciplines, and of patients, audit can build a better picture of the overall effect and contribution of healthcare treatments than is possible from one discipline's perspective. This trend is partially in response to the increasing need to demonstrate improved outcomes and health gain, and also the requirement of the contracting environment, where purchasers and providers need to identify the appropriateness of interventions and approaches for addressing any weaknesses.

Audit criteria relating to cardiac rehabilitation are available following a multidisciplinary consensus workshop held at the Royal College of Physicians in October 1994[20], and can be adapted for use at local level (see Appendix 2).

Outcomes and 'quality-of-life' measures

As more and more interventions are identified, and as debate continues over their appropriateness, it becomes increasingly important to measure outcomes, in order to assess the effectiveness of the interventions concerned. Assessment has been defined as determining how fully and consistently an intervention produces the desired outcome in the patient population for which it was designed[21]. It can be demonstrated that the assessment of outcomes is heavily loaded on the side of hard endpoints, i.e. functional endpoints related to exercise stress testing and symptomatic improvement, and that gaps exist in the areas of quality of life assessment. The American Association of Cardiovascular and Pulmonary Rehabilitation (AACVPR) is addressing outcomes in three areas: health, clinical and behavioural aspects[22]. These include mortality, morbidity, cardiopulmonary function and functional capacity, psychological functioning, risk factor modification, quality of life, social support and return to work.

Physiological measures may provide interesting information to the clinician, but may not be the most relevant concern for the patient. Exercise capacity in an artificial test situation may bear little relation to the patient's capacity to perform activities of daily living, an issue of far greater relevance to the individual. Guyatt[23] describes two approaches to quality-of-life measurement: generic instruments which provide a summary of health-related quality-of-life, and specific instruments which focus on problems associated with single disease states, patient groups or areas of function. Chapter 6 describes some of the quality-of-life measures currently used in the UK, but it is clear that further developmental work is needed in this area. Measures used appropriately can be valid and reliable; used wrongly, they will reinforce the scepticism of those who doubt the potential to quantify such issues. They must therefore be chosen with caution, administered by those with adequate skills and training in their use, and interpreted with care.

Adherence

Oldridge states that as many as 40–50% of patients drop out within 6–12 months of referral to an exercise rehabilitation programme[24]. Motivation specifically related to exercise is discussed in Chapter 5, but the issue of adherence to rehabilitation as a whole is an important one. Poor attendance may be related to a number of factors including psychological factors, environmental and social factors, characteristics of the programme, and the interaction between members of the multidisciplinary team and the participants. The CR programme co-ordinator needs to ensure, in planning service provision, that logistical problems, such as timing of sessions, ease of access to the programme, availability of transport, are not an obstacle to participation. Other issues will need to be addressed in a broader sense, looking at motivation in general, and at assessing each individual for particular factors which may affect them, such as spouse anxiety, perceptions of the importance of health, and a range of socioeconomic factors.

Adequate emergency response

The safety of a programme will depend greatly on adequate planning to reduce or avoid potentially dangerous situations, e.g. screening and risk stratification of patients. In addition to this it is essential to have developed a comprehensive plan of action in the event of an emergency situation. The following points should be considered:

- *All* staff should be certified as competent at Basic Life Support level;
- At least one member of staff involved in the supervision of exercise sessions should be certified as competent in Advanced Cardiac Life Support;
- There should be a policy of regular review and updating the training of *all* staff involved in resuscitation at *all* levels;
- For exercise sessions, a staffing policy should exist which states the ratio of staff to patients.

The AACVPR recommended ratio of staff to patients for immediate outpatient groups (within two weeks of discharge) is 1:5, and for intermediate and maintenance sessions, 1:15[25].

This ratio will be influenced by several factors:

- Range of clinical conditions and the selection process;
- Ratio of high-, moderate- and low-risk patients in each session;
- The physical layout of the environment, including
  - quantity of equipment
  - the type of exercise
  - health and safety regulations in operation;
- Proximity to other sources of assistance.

Such a policy should be strictly implemented even where overall staffing numbers are reduced due to sick leave or other factors, otherwise safety regulations become invalid. Staff must not supervise exercise sessions with unsafe levels of staffing, even though they may feel that they are 'letting the patients down' in a particular instance. The policy should state the action to be taken in the event of staff being unavailable; sessions may have to be cancelled or the numbers of patients and degree of exercise undertaken that day may need to be restricted.

List of key points

- Cardiac rehabilitation should be practised using a multidisciplinary approach.
- Coronary heart disease should be recognized as a chronic disease process, and patients allowed to move freely within the rehabilitation programme according to their individual needs.
- The four phases of cardiac rehabilitation outlined should be set in a flexible time structure.
- Programmes should aim for individual goal-setting incorporating a structure for regular review.
- Safety and effectiveness, and their ongoing evaluation, should be of paramount importance.

References

1. National Forum for Coronary Heart Disease (1994) *Women and Heart Disease*, London: Wordworks.
2. McGee, H.M. and Horgan, J.H. (1992) Cardiac rehabilitation programmes: are women less likely to attend? *British Medical Journal*, **305**, 283–4.
3. Ades, P., Waldmann, M.L., Polk, D.M. and Coflesky, J.T. (1992) Referral patterns and exercise response in the rehabilitation of female coronary patients aged > 62 years. *American Journal of Cardiology*, **69**, 1422–5.
4. Balfour, I.C., Drimmer, A.M., Nouri, S., Pennington, D.G., Hemkens, C.L. and Harvey, L.L. (1991) Paediatric cardiac rehabilitation. *American Journal of Disease in Children*, **145**, 627–30.
5. Personal communication with Mr G.S. Bowman and Professor D.R. Thompson, Institute of Nursing Studies, University of Hull. February 1995.
6. Lewin, B., Robertson, I.H., Cay, E.L. *et al.* (1992) Effects of self-help post-myocardial infarction rehabilitation on psychological adjustment and use of health services. *Lancet*, **339**, 1036–40.
7. Department of Health (1993) *What Seems to be the Matter? Communication between Hospitals and Patients*, London: HMSO.
8. Ben-Ari, E. (1995) Rehabilitation of the cardiac patient during hospitalization: inpatient programs. In: M.L. Pollock and D.H. Schmidt (eds) *Heart Disease and Rehabilitation*, Champaign, Illinois: Human Kinetics Books.
9. Beitman, B.D., Mukerji, V., Flaker, G. and Basha, I.M. (1988) Panic disorder, cardiology patients, and atypical chest pain. *Psychiatric Clinics of North America*, **11**(2): 387–97.
10. American Association of Cardiovascular and Pulmonary Rehabilitation (1995) Documentation. In: *Guidelines for Cardiac Rehabilitation*, 2nd edn Champaign, Illinois: Human Kinetics Books.

11. Thompson, D.R. and Cordle, C.J. (1988) Support of wives of myocardial infarction patients, *Journal of Advanced Nursing*, **13**, 223–8.
12. Girdano, D.A. and Dusek, D.E. (1988) *Changing Health Behaviour*, Scottsdale, Arizona: Gorsuch Scarisbrick.
13. Hansen, M. and Streff, M. (1995) Patient education: practical guidelines. In: M.L. Pollock and D.H. Schmidt (eds), *Heart Disease and Rehabilitation*, Champaign, Illinois: Human Kinetics Books.
14. Laidlaw, J.M. and Harden, R.M. (1987) Printed material for patients with heart disease: Are we really 'educating patients? *Medical Teacher*, **9**, 201–3.
15. Van Camp, S. (1995) Safety, precautions, and emergency procedures. In: M.L. Pollock and D.H. Schmidt (eds), *Heart Disease and Rehabilitation*, Champaign, Illinois: Human Kinetics Books.
16. Executive Committee (1986) *Guidelines for Cardiac Rehabilitation*, Massachusetts Association of Cardiovascular and Pulmonary Rehabilitation.
17. Biddle, S., Fox, K. and Edmunds, L. (1994) *Physical Activity Promotion in Primary Health Care in England*, Exercise and Sport Behaviour Research and Promotion Department, Exeter University.
18. Horgan, J., Bethell, H., Carson, P., Davidson, C., Julian, D., Mayou, R.A. and Nagle, R. (1992) British Cardiac Society Working Party Report on Cardiac Rehabilitation, *British Heart Journal*, **67**, 412–8.
19. Department of Health (1991) *Audit Report: Clinical Audit in the Nursing and Therapy Professions*, London: HMSO.
20. Thompson, D.R., Bowman, G.S., Kitson, A.L., de Bono, D.P. and Hopkins, A. (Submitted for publication 1995) Cardiac Rehabilitation: guidelines and audit standards. Report of a workshop held jointly by the National Institute for Nursing, the Research Unit of the Royal College of Physicians and the British Cardiac Society.
21. Michel, T.H. (1992) Outcome assessment in cardiac rehabilitation, *International Journal of Technological Assessment in Health Care*, **8**, 76–84.
22. Herbert, W.G.(1994) The outcomes 'movement' in health care: causes and consequences for cardiac rehabilitation, *Exercise Standards and Malpractice Reporter*, **8(5)**, 65–79.
23. Guyatt, G.H., Feeny, D.H. and Patrick, D.L. (1993) Measuring health related quality of life, *Annals of Internal Medicine*, **118**, 622–29.
24. Oldridge, N.B., Donner, A.P., Buck, C.W., Jones, N.L., Andrew, G.M., Parker, J.O., Cunningham, D.A., Kavaknach, T., Rechnitzer, P.A. and Sutton, J.R. (1983) Predictors of dropout from cardiac exercise rehabilitation: Ontario Collaborative Exercise-Heart Study, *American Journal of Cardiology*, **51**, 70–4.
25. American Association of Cardiovascular and Pulmonary Rehabilitation (1995) Personnel for rehabilitation services, In *Guidelines for Cardiac Rehabilitation*, 2nd edn Champaign, Illinois: Human Kinetics Books.

Recommended reading

American Association of Cardiovascular and Pulmonary Rehabilitation (1995)
Guidelines for Cardiac Rehabilitation (2nd edn)
Champaign, Illinois: Human Kinetics Books.

Hall, L. (ed.) (1993)
Developing and Managing Cardiac Rehabilitation Programs
Champaign, Illinois: Human Kinetics Books.

Jones, D. and West, R. (eds) 1995
Cardiac Rehabilitation
London, BMJ Publishing Group.

Pollock, M.L. and Schmidt, D.H. (eds) (1995)
Heart Disease and Rehabilitation (3rd edn)
Champaign, Illinois: Human Kinetics Books.

Sharp, I. (ed.) (1994)
Coronary Heart Disease: Are Women Special?
London: National Forum for Coronary Heart Disease Prevention.

Thompson, D.R., Bowman, G.S., Kitson, A.L., de Bono, D.P. and Hopkins, A. (1995)
Cardiac Rehabilitation: Guidelines and Audit Standards.
Report of a workshop held jointly by the National Institute for Nursing, the Research Unit of the Royal College of Physicians and the British Cardiac Society. (Submitted for publication)

Wenger, N. and Hellerstein, H. (1992)
Rehabilitation of the Coronary Patient (3rd edn)
New York: Churchill Livingstone.

Programme documentation

Hospital setting
Cardiac Rehabilitation Co-ordinator
Department of Cardiology
Beaumont Hospital
Dublin 9
Ireland

Community setting
Cardiac Rehabilitation Co-ordinator
The Basingstoke and Alton Cardiac Rehabilitation Unit
Alton Health Centre
Anstey Road
Alton
Hants GU34 2QX

Chapter 3

Medical Aspects of Cardiac Rehabilitation

Summary

The purpose of this chapter is to describe medical aspects of cardiac rehabilitation. Readers will be referred to key works for further information on relevant issues.

Medical goals

Introduction

Patients with coronary heart disease (CHD) can derive major medical benefits from participation in cardiac rehabilitation (CR) programmes. These benefits include: an increase in anginal threshold; an increase in exercise tolerance; a reduction in the need for anti-anginal and antihypertensive medication; an improvement in lipid profiles and clotting profiles, and improvements in other risk factors, such as insulin resistance. These are all in addition to the improvements in psychological function and quality of life. There has also been strong evidence from overviews of CR programmes that there may be an overall reduction in mortality achieved by participation in a CR programme incorporating an exercise training element. The two important overviews of CR[1,2] have shown that, despite variability between small trials, the overall effect of participation in CR is for a net reduction in mortality of approximately 25% (which was statistically significant).

The mechanism of benefit is unclear but sceptics of the benefits of such programmes tend to attribute such improvements to improved surveillance of cardiac patients. If this is so, then it emphasizes the importance of good medical practice in the patient's management. Increased patient contact with healthcare personnel is likely to improve the chances of appropriate management of medical problems which could otherwise jeopardize the patient's chance of survival.

Patients with CHD are subject to sudden deterioration – even when seemingly clinically stable – and prompt institution of appropriate therapy is often important. Additionally, the regular assessment and modification of therapy for other vascular conditions such as hypertension which have an impact on both coronary event risk and indirectly related conditions such as stroke, is likely to be beneficial.

The medical goals of CR have been summarized by the World Health Organization as follows[3]:

- The prevention of cardiac death;
- A decrease in cardiac morbidity, e.g. reduced incidence of myocardial infarction (MI) and coronary artery bypass graft (CABG) closure;
- Relief of symptoms such as angina and breathlessness.

The medical input required to achieve these goals can be conveniently considered under four headings:

- Risk stratification;
- Further diagnostic testing and intervention;
- Therapeutics including risk factor modification;
- Programme management, efficacy, and logistics.

Risk stratification

It is known that mortality after a first myocardial infarction depends on several variables, of which the most important is the size of the index infarct[4]. A wide variety of non-invasive testing measures can predict additional risk. Problems such as early recurrent ischaemia with risk of re-infarction, additional coronary artery stenoses in vessels other than the vessel of the index infarct, and risk of arrhythmia, can be predicted from multiple methods of assessment. Unfortunately, the positive predictive value of most of these tests is poor. The negative predictive value however is high[5]. This means that a patient without demonstrated complications from the index infarct, with good effort tolerance and freedom from evidence of ischaemia, symptoms and ventricular impairment, will do well and remain at low risk, often for a number of years[6]. Cardiac rehabilitation programmes often include such patients, many of whom are also motivated to modify the risk factors which contributed to their disease originally. It is difficult in such a patient to demonstrate that the programme enhances likelihood of long-term survival.

In the UK, risk stratification is most commonly performed by exercise electrocardiography alone, although additional prognostic information may be obtained by radionuclide perfusion imaging combined with functional testing[7]. The post-infarction electrocardiogram presents difficulties of interpretation during exercise[8]. Routine radionuclide study would probably be impossible for all post-MI patients in the UK. The majority of CR programmes use exercise elec-trocardiogram (ECG) testing not only as an aid to find the patient who requires further evaluation by coronary angiography or who is unsuitable at that point in time for inclusion, but also to determine exercise prescription, which should be individualized for each patient[9].

Controversy exists over even this aspect of the medical screening process. Early exercise testing may pick up the patient with important recurrent myocardial ischaemia. Later, often higher intensity, testing may identify additional patients at risk[10]. Exercise prescription is best made with the patient on the long-term treatment of choice (e.g. beta-blockade). Treatment with such drugs may mask ischaemia, although there is evidence that ischaemia which is evident while on treatment is of more serious prognostic significance[11]. Pragmatism dictates that exercise testing while on therapy is valuable.

Recently the concept of exercise testing following MI treated with thrombolytic drugs has been challenged[12]. Presumably there is considerable hazard in the short-term from the patent but still stenosed coronary artery. There is evidence that thrombolysed patients demonstrate a higher re-occlusion rate over the next three years than non-thrombolysed patients but this does not explain why the mortality curves in thrombolytic studies do not converge as time goes on[13]. The risk of re-closure may then depend on haemostatic variables which are unpredictable, at least by exercise testing. Such assertions, however, are usually made after exam-ination of short-term follow-up data. One of the strongest predictors of long-term risk remains the number of coronary vessels diseased[8]. It is likely that some form of functional assessment will remain the cornerstone of techniques designed to identify the patients at greatest risk, especially as both left ventricular function and exercise capacity are additionally predictive of outcome.

Whatever technique is applied to the assessment of the post-MI patient, or the patient with coronary artery disease in general, the interaction of CR personnel with the patient and the physician responsible for the patient's care is likely to remain important in determining optimum therapy for the patient.

Further diagnostic testing and intervention

Coronary angiography has been proposed as the appropriate further investiga-tion in the majority (probably about 80%) of post-MI patients. Although this policy, advocated by Kulick and Rahimtoola[8], is not practical in the UK, it is important to examine the possible advantages which such an approach may confer. Although coronary angiography combined with left ventriculography can enhance diagnostic precision, it can be argued that only patients with operable three-vessel coronary artery disease or left main coronary artery disease definitely benefit in terms of survival from coronary surgery. Given the likely benefits in terms of symptoms, a wider range of patients is likely to obtain some benefit from surgery. The significance of a severe residual stenosis in the infarct-related artery is still debated, and trials designed to determine possible benefit of intervention for such disease, such as Thrombolysis In Myocardial Infarction (TIMI IIB) and Should We Intervene Following Thrombolysis (SWIFT), did not demonstrate any utility of routinely re-vascularizing such lesions[14,15]. From the point of view of the rehabilitation patient however, the value of such an approach lies in the optimization of the patient's risk before even entering the CR programme. The early exercise assessment, and the additional surveillance of CR staff in the early phases of an inpatient or outpatient programme, may help to identify the patient who needs invasive investigation.

Re-vascularization by CABG or by PTCA is continuously improving from the technical standpoint. Recent overviews of long-term results of CABG confirm that a clear difference exists between the fate of medically treated patients with left main coronary artery stenosis and three-vessel disease[16] and that of those treated surgically. Although these results were principally obtained in symptomatic patients it seems reasonable to generalize them to asymptomatic patients following MI. In addition, despite their generally better prognosis, patients with double- and single-vessel disease are also likely to benefit from intervention when the disease subtends a large volume of myocardium. Proximal disease of the left anterior descending coronary artery is important and may also require re-vascularization[17] although such patients were consistently excluded from randomization to surgery or medical therapy in the Coronary Artery Surgery Study (CASS)[18].

Therapeutics and risk factor modification

Skilled use of drug therapy probably contributes substantially to the benefits which accrue to the patient in a CR programme. This area of medical treatment also lends itself readily to relatively simple but powerful methods of audit. For example, a number of publications demonstrate the lack of use of drugs with proven efficacy in the post-MI patient[19]. This has been demonstrated for beta-blocking drugs, and it is highly likely that many patients who could benefit from angiotensin-converting enzyme (ACE)-inhibitors are similarly not receiving this therapy. On the other hand, the uptake of drugs which have almost universal applicability in patients with CHD, such as aspirin, is probably much better.

The conditions amenable to recognition and treatment during cardiac follow-up include:

- Angina pectoris
- Cardiac arrhythmias
- Cardiac failure
- Hyperlipidaemia and dyslipidaemia
- Hypertension
- Transient ischaemic attacks
- Diabetes mellitus

- Hyperuricaemia
- Drug toxicity and side-effects.

As discussed in the Introduction, the appropriate therapy and reassessment of treatment efficacy within a CR programme is likely to reduce long-term risk. Modification of risk factors, although difficult, is enhanced by multiple contacts between patient and therapist. This has been particularly well demonstrated for cigarette smoking, where regular reinforcement improves efficacy of a smoking cessation programme[20]. In the case of cigarette smoking this is also a risk factor where there is clear evidence of benefit in patients who can stop smoking after an MI[21].

Many patients with CHD will demonstrate what is termed 'dyslipidaemia', i.e. a poor profile of plasma high-density lipoprotein and low-density lipoprotein cholesterol and triglyceride. This is to distinguish such patients from the definite 'hyperlipidaemic' patient, usually with heterozygous familial hypercholesterolaemia, where there will be little controversy over the need for treatment. Moderate degrees of lipid abnormality may still carry an adverse prognosis in the patient with manifest coronary artery disease. There is increasing evidence that intervention with strict diet and/or lipid-lowering drugs can produce both atheroma regression and a reduction in long-term mortality. There is a considerable potential for staff of a CR programme to have an impact on this risk factor[22,23,26] (see Chapter 7).

Other newer risk factors continue to be described. Fibrinogen levels is one of the most powerful predictors of risk in the post-MI patient. On the other hand there is no intervention other than smoking cessation, and possibly fairly vigorous exercise which influences this particularly[24,25]. Further research will reveal whether any drug-based approach will be of value in patients with high fibrinogen levels.

Cardiac rehabilitation needs to be conducted against the background of continuing medical surveillance and the management of other conditions. An extremely brief summary of common medical management of some of these follows.

Hyperlipidaemia

Lipid reduction is an important aspect of treating patients with CHD, and involves lifestyle modifications and particularly dietary advice. In patients with persistently raised cholesterol levels, drug treatment is sometimes necessary. The results of the important Scandinavian Simvastatin Survival Study (4S)[26] has already shown that in patients with CHD, reduction in cholesterol to below 5.5 mmol/l leads to a dramatic reduction in mortality of the order of 40% or more. The effect is slow to develop, and the survival curves separate after six months or longer. It should be stressed, therefore, that all patients with CHD should have their lipid profile measured routinely, and any person whose cholesterol remains

■ Hyperuricaemia
■ Drug toxicity and side-effects.

As discussed in the Introduction, the appropriate therapy and reassessment of treatment efficacy within a CR programme is likely to reduce long-term risk. Modification of risk factors, although difficult, is enhanced by multiple contacts between patient and therapist. This has been particularly well demonstrated for cigarette smoking, where regular reinforcement improves efficacy of a smoking cessation programme[20]. In the case of cigarette smoking this is also a risk factor where there is clear evidence of benefit in patients who can stop smoking after an MI[21].

Many patients with CHD will demonstrate what is termed 'dyslipidaemia', i.e. a poor profile of plasma high-density lipoprotein and low-density lipoprotein cholesterol and triglyceride. This is to distinguish such patients from the definite 'hyperlipidaemic' patient, usually with heterozygous familial hypercholesterolaemia, where there will be little controversy over the need for treatment. Moderate degrees of lipid abnormality may still carry an adverse prognosis in the patient with manifest coronary artery disease. There is increasing evidence that intervention with strict diet and/or lipid-lowering drugs can produce both atheroma regression and a reduction in long-term mortality. There is a considerable potential for staff of a CR programme to have an impact on this risk factor[22,23,26] (see Chapter 7).

Other newer risk factors continue to be described. Fibrinogen levels is one of the most powerful predictors of risk in the post-MI patient. On the other hand there is no intervention other than smoking cessation, and possibly fairly vigorous exercise which influences this particularly[24,25]. Further research will reveal whether any drug-based approach will be of value in patients with high fibrinogen levels.

Cardiac rehabilitation needs to be conducted against the background of continuing medical surveillance and the management of other conditions. An extremely brief summary of common medical management of some of these follows.

Hyperlipidaemia

Lipid reduction is an important aspect of treating patients with CHD, and involves lifestyle modifications and particularly dietary advice. In patients with persistently raised cholesterol levels, drug treatment is sometimes necessary. The results of the important Scandinavian Simvastatin Survival Study (4S)[26] has already shown that in patients with CHD, reduction in cholesterol to below 5.5 mmol/l leads to a dramatic reduction in mortality of the order of 40% or more. The effect is slow to develop, and the survival curves separate after six months or longer. It should be stressed, therefore, that all patients with CHD should have their lipid profile measured routinely, and any person whose cholesterol remains

Patients with CHD are subject to sudden deterioration – even when seemingly clinically stable – and prompt institution of appropriate therapy is often important. Additionally, the regular assessment and modification of therapy for other vascular conditions such as hypertension which have an impact on both coronary event risk and indirectly related conditions such as stroke, is likely to be beneficial.

The medical goals of CR have been summarized by the World Health Organization as follows[3]:

■ The prevention of cardiac death;
■ A decrease in cardiac morbidity, e.g. reduced incidence of myocardial infarction (MI) and coronary artery bypass graft (CABG) closure;
■ Relief of symptoms such as angina and breathlessness.

The medical input required to achieve these goals can be conveniently considered under four headings:

■ Risk stratification;
■ Further diagnostic testing and intervention;
■ Therapeutics including risk factor modification;
■ Programme management, efficacy, and logistics.

Risk stratification

It is known that mortality after a first myocardial infarction depends on several variables, of which the most important is the size of the index infarct[4]. A wide variety of non-invasive testing measures can predict additional risk. Problems such as early recurrent ischaemia with risk of re-infarction, additional coronary artery stenoses in vessels other than the vessel of the index infarct, and risk of arrhythmia, can be predicted from multiple methods of assessment. Unfortunately, the positive predictive value of most of these tests is poor. The negative predictive value however is high[5]. This means that a patient without demonstrated complications from the index infarct, with good effort tolerance and freedom from evidence of ischaemia, symptoms and ventricular impairment, will do well and remain at low risk, often for a number of years[6]. Cardiac rehabilitation programmes often include such patients, many of whom are also motivated to modify the risk factors which contributed to their disease originally. It is difficult in such a patient to demonstrate that the programme enhances likelihood of long-term survival.

In the UK, risk stratification is most commonly performed by exercise electrocardiography alone, although additional prognostic information may be obtained by radionuclide perfusion imaging combined with functional testing[7]. The post-infarction electrocardiogram presents difficulties of interpretation during exercise[8]. Routine radionuclide study would probably be impossible for all post-MI patients in the UK. The majority of CR programmes use exercise electrocardiogram (ECG) testing not only as an aid to find the patient who requires further evaluation by coronary angiography or who is unsuitable at that point in time for inclusion, but also to determine exercise prescription, which should be individualized for each patient[9].

Controversy exists over even this aspect of the medical screening process. Early exercise testing may pick up the patient with important recurrent myocardial ischaemia. Later, often higher intensity, testing may identify additional patients at risk[10]. Exercise prescription is best made with the patient on the long-term treatment of choice (e.g. beta-blockade). Treatment with such drugs may mask ischaemia, although there is evidence that ischaemia which is evident while on treatment is of more serious prognostic significance[11]. Pragmatism dictates that exercise testing while on therapy is valuable.

Recently the concept of exercise testing following MI treated with thrombolytic drugs has been challenged[12]. Presumably there is considerable hazard in the short-term from the patent but still stenosed coronary artery. There is evidence that thrombolysed patients demonstrate a higher re-occlusion rate over the next three years than non-thrombolysed patients but this does not explain why the mortality curves in thrombolytic studies do not converge as time goes on[13]. The risk of re-closure may then depend on haemostatic variables which are unpredictable, at least by exercise testing. Such assertions, however, are usually made after examination of short-term follow-up data. One of the strongest predictors of long-term risk remains the number of coronary vessels diseased[8]. It is likely that some form of functional assessment will remain the cornerstone of techniques designed to identify the patients at greatest risk, especially as both left ventricular function and exercise capacity are additionally predictive of outcome.

Whatever technique is applied to the assessment of the post-MI patient, or the patient with coronary artery disease in general, the interaction of CR personnel with the patient and the physician responsible for the patient's care is likely to remain important in determining optimum therapy for the patient.

Further diagnostic testing and intervention

Coronary angiography has been proposed as the appropriate further investigation in the majority (probably about 80%) of post-MI patients. Although this policy, advocated by Kulick and Rahimtoola[8], is not practical in the UK, it is important to examine the possible advantages which such an approach may confer. Although coronary angiography combined with left ventriculography can enhance diagnostic precision, it can be argued that only patients with operable three-vessel coronary artery disease or left main coronary artery disease definitely benefit in terms of survival from coronary surgery. Given the likely benefits in terms of symptoms, a wider range of patients is likely to obtain some benefit from surgery. The significance of a severe residual stenosis in the infarct-related artery is still debated, and trials designed to determine possible benefit of intervention

for such disease, such as Thrombolysis In Myocardial Infarction (TIMI IIB) and Should We Intervene Following Thrombolysis (SWIFT), did not demonstrate any utility of routinely re-vascularizing such lesions[14,15]. From the point of view of the rehabilitation patient however, the value of such an approach lies in the optimization of the patient's risk before even entering the CR programme. The early exercise assessment, and the additional surveillance of CR staff in the early phases of an inpatient or outpatient programme, may help to identify the patient who needs invasive investigation.

Re-vascularization by CABG or by PTCA is continuously improving from the technical standpoint. Recent overviews of long-term results of CABG confirm that a clear difference exists between the fate of medically treated patients with left main coronary artery stenosis and three-vessel disease[16] and that of those treated surgically. Although these results were principally obtained in symptomatic patients it seems reasonable to generalize them to asymptomatic patients following MI. In addition, despite their generally better prognosis, patients with double- and single-vessel disease are also likely to benefit from intervention when the disease subtends a large volume of myocardium. Proximal disease of the left anterior descending coronary artery is important and may also require re-vascularization[17] although such patients were consistently excluded from randomization to surgery or medical therapy in the Coronary Artery Surgery Study (CASS)[18].

Therapeutics and risk factor modification

Skilled use of drug therapy probably contributes substantially to the benefits which accrue to the patient in a CR programme. This area of medical treatment also lends itself readily to relatively simple but powerful methods of audit. For example, a number of publications demonstrate the lack of use of drugs with proven efficacy in the post-MI patient[19]. This has been demonstrated for beta-blocking drugs, and it is highly likely that many patients who could benefit from angiotensin-converting enzyme (ACE)-inhibitors are similarly not receiving this therapy. On the other hand, the uptake of drugs which have almost universal applicability in patients with CHD, such as aspirin, is probably much better.

The conditions amenable to recognition and treatment during cardiac follow-up include:

- Angina pectoris
- Cardiac arrhythmias
- Cardiac failure
- Hyperlipidaemia and dyslipidaemia
- Hypertension
- Transient ischaemic attacks
- Diabetes mellitus

above 5.5 mmol/l despite dietary intervention should be considered for treatment with a 'statin' drug, or an alternative agent where the lipid profile so dictates.

Hypertension

The evidence for the benefits of medical treatment of raised blood pressure is beyond doubt for moderate and severe hypertension[27]. The situation for mild hypertension is less clear-cut in terms of overall mortality, and any cut-off value of blood pressure above which treatment is recommended will inevitably be arbitrary. However, the evidence for the benefit of reducing high blood pressure as a risk factor in patients after MI is stronger, because of the greater chance these patients will eventually develop a coronary related morbid or mortal event. In particular, the use of beta-blockers or ACE inhibitors in this situation is to be recommended. The benefits of treating hypertension in the elderly population has also been shown to be particularly effective at reducing the occurrence of both MI and cerebrovascular events, and in this age group the use of thiazide diuretics in particular appears to be beneficial[28-30].

Transient ischaemic attacks

Transient ischaemic attacks (TIAs) can be caused by carotid arterial disease, and where severe, can be improved by carotid surgery. In addition, regular aspirin (usually a dose of 300 mg or 600 mg daily) significantly reduces the incidence of TIAs and prevents more major strokes. The vast majority of patients with CHD will have already been recommended to take aspirin, although the treatment of TIAs usually requires the use of a slightly higher dose. Anticoagulation is sometimes recommended where TIAs persist despite treatment with aspirin. Where both carotid and coronary surgery is required in the same patient it may be logical to undertake the surgery at the same time, if local facilities so allow.

Diabetes

The management of diabetes mellitus is essential in maintaining the quality and quantity of the lives of patients affected with this condition. In the presence of diabetes and CHD, and any other associated features, such as renal impairment and hypertension, the degree of care taken in respect of management is recommended to be even greater than for other high-risk patients without diabetes. The targets may be different, such as the need for keeping blood pressure down to lower levels than is usually recommended for non-diabetic patients. For example, it has been recommended that the blood pressure be kept to below 130/85 rather than more common levels of 140 or 150/90 or 95 for patients without diabetes. There is also evidence that the use of ACE inhibitors can delay renal impairment progression in patients with diabetes due to the reduction in the rate of proteinuria.

Hyperuricaemia

Although raised uric acid levels are associated with increased risk of CHD, as yet there is no definitive evidence that reducing these pharmacologically with, for example, allopurinol, leads to any reduction in the severity or progression of CHD. It may, however, lead to a reduction in the rate of attacks of gout, but of course the possibility that acute institution of allopurinol could lead to precipitation of attacks of gout should always be borne in mind.

Cardiac rehabilitation in special patient groups

The benefits and risks of taking part in a CR programme after an MI depend on the prior morbidity and prognosis of the individual. The lower the cardiovascular risk, and the better the exercise tolerance and state of health of the patient at the start, then the lower the chance of any adverse events occurring during the CR programme. These low-risk patients, however, may have less to gain from rehabilitation if their degree of fitness and motivation are already high. By contrast, patients at higher risk of re-infarction, or with a lower level of motivation and exercise tolerance may achieve more substantial benefit from rehabilitation. Where resources are limited, the selection of participants in rehabilitation is important to maximize the benefits of the programme. It is a valid criticism that CR may be offered more to the lower risk younger patient than the higher risk older patients with more medical problems. Although there are more complications and difficulties with recruiting complicated, elderly or high-risk patients into the CR programme, even modest reductions in risk factors and improvements in exercise tolerance may be of substantial benefit to these patients. It should be emphasized that even where patients may not be able to participate fully in the exercise component, for reasons described in the following sections, they should not be excluded from a CR programme altogether as there is much to be gained from other equally important factors, such as lifestyle change and stress management components[31].

Older patients

An effective age restriction often exists for many CR programmes. Physiologically and medically there is no reason for age *per se* to be a contraindication to rehabilitation. The risk factors for cardiovascular disease may differ in the elderly, with dyslipidaemia and hyperlipidaemia being quantitatively less important, and systolic blood pressure being more important, but there can still be advantage in identifying and reducing these risk factors. Exercise tolerance is more markedly impaired at outset, but even in the very elderly it can be increased by training. Other diseases frequently co-exist, including chronic lung diseases, senile cardiac fibrosis, conduction system disease, arthritis, muscle weakness and osteoporosis.

These and many other factors make CR programmes with an exercise component more problematic, and associated with a higher rate of complications. This does not mean, however, that the benefits may not still over-ride the risks.

The elderly are likely to need a more graded introduction to CR, more frequent and prolonged contact throughout the programme, and closer attention from medical staff. These patients will often present with other non-cardiac problems requiring assistance from a range of medical specialities and other health professionals. It is wise to incorporate these professionals in the CR visits of the elderly patient so that there is no conflict of advice about management of daily activities and lifestyle advice. The benefits of recruiting more elderly patients can be very important in helping this group to achieve a greater degree of independence, thus avoiding the need for additional services including long-term residential care.

Angina

The management of angina aims to improve exercise tolerance and reduce the frequency of anginal episodes. The main pharmacological treatments include aspirin plus beta-blockers, and long- and short-acting nitrates, supplemented where appropriate by calcium antagonists, and the newer potassium channel openers. The choice for a particular drug group depends on other patient factors, including the presence of other illnesses which might affect the response to a drug, or contraindications to particular agents, such as asthma being a contraindication for the use of beta-blockers.

Some patients with residual coronary artery stenoses may manifest episodes of ST-segment depression on ECG monitoring, which could represent silent episodes of myocardial ischaemia. It is not certain, so far, from the available evidence whether there is a need to treat these episodes specifically, although most anti-anginal medications will also reduce the frequency of the 'silent episodes'.

Continuing, or unstable, angina frequently prevents a patient from participating in a formal exercise programme. Participation can be delayed until completion of further investigation and re-vascularization procedures where these are being contemplated, but there remains a substantial population of patients with persistent angina in whom re-vascularization procedures are either not possible or incompletely successful. These patients may gain benefit in terms of secondary prevention and in improving exercise tolerance by participating in a programme. There is good evidence for a modest anti-anginal effect of physical training, and in addition risk factor reduction is of considerable importance for angina patients[32]. Training in the presence of exercise-induced angina may also actually promote the development of new collateral vessels to the myocardium. Modification of anti-anginal therapy might allow a greater exercise tolerance so that patients can more fully participate in the exercise component of a CR programme.

From a practical point of view there are increased difficulties for the patient with regular anginal attacks participating in an exercise programme. There is probably an important, albeit unquantified, extra risk associated with exercise in people with regular anginal attacks during exercise. The angina may interfere with the ability of the patients to perform sufficient exercise to gain a training effect, and there are the practical difficulties associated with patients experiencing bouts of angina during exercise sessions. Where the anginal threshold is stable and predictable, an exercise regimen can be designed to train the patient at sub-anginal exercise intensities. There is also an opportunity for greater supervision of these patients which would assist in the evaluation of their possible need for further medical intervention.

Cardiac arrhythmias

With the exception of atrial fibrillation and life-threatening episodes of ventricular tachycardia (VT), most cardiac arrhythmias do not require specific treatment unless they cause symptomatic deterioration. It is now known that over-zealous treatment of recurrent bouts of ventricular ectopics, or non-sustained episodes of ventricular tachycardia which did not produce symptoms, may be likely to increase mortality rather than reduce it. This was shown in the important Cardiac Arrhythmia Suppression Trial (CAST) study[33]. Only where symptomatic deterioration is associated with runs of ventricular tachycardia is it mandatory to commence anti-arrhythmic therapy, and the choice of agent will depend on other patient factors. The best safety profile in terms of a lower incidence of pro-arrhythmic episodes is probably gained by using amiodarone, although its list of potential side-effects is quite large.

Other arrhythmias can be treated with symptomatic improvement and improvement in objective measures of left ventricular function and exercise performance. These include atrial fibrillation and flutter, and paroxysmal supraventricular tachycardias.

Bradyarrhythmias can be treated with pacemakers, and consideration should be given to the use of more sophisticated pacemakers, such as dual chamber pacing with rate responsiveness. These can improve exercise tolerance in patients with left ventricular impairment, or with a very poor heart rate response to exercise.

Cardiac failure

The medical management of cardiac failure has undergone major changes over the last ten years. There have been documented major improvements in exercise performance and survival with the treatment of patients of heart failure, with angiotensin-converting-enzyme (ACE)-inhibitors at all stages of the evolution of this syndrome. It is now recommended that all patients with significant left ventricular impairment (such as would be seen after a large anterior MI) should recieve treatment with ACE-inhibitors regardless of whether they manifest cardiac failure or not. In addition, all patients with cardiac failue of any severity should be offered the opportunity to improve with ACE-inhibitors, but there is a small group with predominantly diastolic dysfunction leading to heart failure, who may not respond so well to ACE-inhibitors. Diuretics remain the mainstay of the treatment of fluid retention and congestion in cardiac failure patients. In patients with atrial fibrillation and a rapid ventricular response, digoxin is beneficial. The routine use of digoxin in heart failure patients in stable sinus rhythm is not recommended in the UK, although results of new trials testing this strategy will be available in the next couple of years. As yet, there has been no convincing evidence of benefit with calcium antagonists in cardiac failure, and there has been some evidence of deterioration in left ventricular function with some of these agents. The combination of nitrates with hydralazine, although shown to be superior to placebo, is less effective than ACE-inhibitors. The use of chronic oral positive inotropic agents has been associated with an increased mortality due to pro-arrythmic effects and is not recommended.

In the past heart failure was frequently listed as an absolute contraindication to participation in CR. Whilst active myocarditis or acute heart failure with congestion remain contraindications to exercise training, research over the last decade has shown that carefully selected cases with stable chronic heart failure can achieve significant and worthwhile benefits from exercise training[34,35]. This is now an important area in CR research. Like the situation for the elderly, these patients are significantly limited and in need of considerable medical care. They are also likely to benefit substantially from even modest improvements in their ability to perform exercise as many daily tasks will stress them close to their cardiopulmonary exercise reserve. These patients are frequently well motivated and co-operate fully with the CR programme[36]. Several practical difficulties arise, however, including the need for closer supervision, more detailed pre-participation assessment, and a greater likelihood of complications, including serious ventricular arrhythmias. Perhaps most importantly from a practical point of view, these patients may need a life-long attachment to the programme for continuing benefit.

Research in specialist units has shown possible training benefits for patients with moderate and severe heart failure provided their condition is stable. Improvements of 20–25% have been seen in exercise capacity associated with reduced sympathetic tone, reduced breathlessness and exercise ventilation, and improved exercise haemodynamics.

However, the training exercise needs to be specially tailored to these patients' reduced capacity. The level of exercise prescription may start at a very low level, such as 60–70% of their existing maximal capacity for as little as 5-10 minutes a session. This is then gradually increased in duration and absolute intensity as the patient's maximal capacity increases.

It is recommended that patients with heart failure perform a cardiopulmonary exercise assessment in a specialist unit to establish accurately their capacity prior to entry. More detailed evaluation will be needed detection of ventricular arrhythmias either on 24-hour ECG mc exercise testing. The presence of ventricular tachycardia is common in patients with moderate and severe heart failure, and may increase the risk of exercise. Whether these arrhythmias negate possible benefits of rehabilitation because of the risk of precipitating arrhythmias remains unknown.

No patient with heart failure should take part in the exercise programme in the presence of acute decompensation such as with pulmonary or peripheral oedema, active myocarditis or febrile illness. Although there is no lower limit on ejection fraction for the participation of patients with heart failure, the patients must be comfortable at rest, and be able to exercise for 5 minutes at an exercise level of 2 metabolic equivalents (METS) or greater. A left ventricular ejection fraction of 20% or less is still compatible with participation, and patients can still usefully participate when stable on a cardiac transplantation waiting list.

Programme management, efficacy and logistics

A clinician who maintains a major commitment to the CR programme is important. Such a clinician will determine the attention paid to the various aspects of the programme according to the latest medical evidence and demonstrated therapeutic efficacy. For example, such a clinician may wish to set protocols for the measurement of, and intervention by, drug therapy for elevated plasma lipids. Since problems are sometimes experienced by programme staff in implementing treatment or in investigation of programme participants, it is important for the clinician to be able to act as the mediator when other medical staff need to be consulted about the patients. A variety of other staff contribute usefully to CR programmes as discussed in Chapter 2. If the programme is run by a programme director or co-ordinator, then this person needs regular contact with the lead clinician.

The efficacy of the programme can be determined by a number of measures which can also be considered as audit standards. A comprehensive list of these is found in the American Association of Cardiovascular and Pulmonary Rehabilitation (AACVPR) Guidelines[9], but a suggested list more appropriate for the UK can be found in Appendix 2.

In the UK, the range of facilities is so wide and the personnel involved with CR so varied that the exact format by which the programme is run cannot be specified (see Chapter 2). Certain minimum standards however should be attained. These are that:

- *All* staff involved with cardiac patients in rehabilitation should have basic life support training;
- If no medical staff are present at any exercise session, then at least one of the staff members present should be trained in advanced life support, of which the most important component is being able to recognize and defibrillate ventricular fibrillation;

- Exercise sessions which are not supervised by medical staff should not include 'high risk' patients (however these are specified by the lead clinician and programme director);
- Exercise sessions during Phase Three of rehabilitation for low-risk patients (the organized outpatient training sessions) should have rapid access to a member of medical staff even if one is not present during the training sessions;
- Drills should be held at intervals to rehearse procedures for management of cardiac arrest and a record book should be kept;
- Involvement of a Resuscitation Training Officer with the programme is beneficial. High risk patients should be offered the option of cardiopulmonary resuscitation training for their spouse or partner or close relatives;
- Adequate record keeping of counselling and training sessions should be in place. Documentation of progress should be made. Other parameters as dictated by research and audit protocols should be recorded;
- Equipment used should be registered under any asset registration schemes and adequate and documented servicing and safety assessments made.

Summary of key points

- CR can improve prognosis and quality of life in a wide variety of patients with CHD.
- The CR programme also involves close attention to modern treatment of other cardiovascular and non-cardiovascular conditions that individual patients suffer.
- Clinical staff need to take an active and collaborative role in all aspects of the CR programme.
- Medical and rehabilitation management should be considered together and the structure of a programme should take this requirement into account.

References

1. Oldridge, N.B., Guyatt, G.H., Fischer, M.E. and Rimm, A.A. (1988) Cardiac rehabilitation after myocardial infarction: Combined experience of randomized clinical trials, *Journal of the American Medical Association*, **260**, 945–50.
2. O'Connor, G.T., Buring, J.E, Yusuf, S., Goldhaber, S.Z., Olmstead, E.M., Paffenbarger, R.S. and Hennekens, C.H. (1989) An overview of randomised controlled trials of rehabilitation with exercise after myocardial infarction, *Circulation*, **80**, 234–44.

3. World Health Organization (1993) *Needs and Action Priorities in Cardiac Rehabilitation and Secondary Prevention in Patients with Coronary Heart Disease*. Geneva: WHO Regional Office for Europe.
4. The Multicenter Postinfarction Research Group (1983) Risk stratification and survival after myocardial infarction, *New England Journal of Medicine*, **309**, 331–6.
5. Northridge, D.B. and Hall, R.J.C. (1994) Post-myocardial infarction exercise testing in the thrombolytic era, *Lancet*, **343**, 1175–6.
6. Campbell, S., A'Hern, R., Quigley, P., Vincent, R., Jewitt, D. and Chamberlain, D. (1988) Identification of patients at low risk of dying after acute myocardial infarction by simple clinical and submaximal exercise test criteria, *European Heart Journal*, **9**, 938–47.
7. Gibson, R.S. and Watson, D.D. (1991) Value of planar[201]Tl imaging in risk stratification of patients recovering from acute myocardial infarction, *Circulation*, **84 (Suppl I)**, I148–62.
8. Kulick, D.L. and Rahimtoola, S.H. (1991) Risk stratification in survivors of acute myocardial infarction: routine cardiac catheterization and angiography is a reasonable approach in most patients, *American Heart Journal*, **121**, 641–56.
9. American Association of Cardiovascular and Pulmonary Rehabilitation (1991) *Guidelines for Cardiac Rehabilitation Programs*, Champaign, Illinois: Human Kinetics Books.
10. Starling, M.R., Crawford, M.H., Kennedy, G.T. and O'Rourke, R.A. (1981) Treadmill exercise tests predischarge and six weeks post-myocardial infarction to detect abnormalities of known prognostic value, *Annals of Internal Medicine*, **94**, 721–7.
11. Mark, D.B., Shaw, L., Harrell, F.E. Jr., Hlatky, M.A., Lee, K.L., Bengtson, J.R., McCants, C.B., *et al.* (1991) Prognostic value of a treadmill exercise score in outpatients with suspected coronary artery disease, *New England Journal of Medicine*, **325**, 849–53.
12. Flapan, A.D. (1994) Management of patients after their first myocardial infarction, *British Medical Journal*, **309**, 1129–34.
13. Simoons, M.L., Vos, J., Tijssen, J.G.P., Vermeer, F., Verheugt, F.W.A., Krauss, X.H. and Manger Cats, V. (1989) Long-term benefit of early thrombolytic therapy in patients with acute myocardial infarction: 5 year follow-up of a trial conducted by the Interuniversity Cardiology Institute of the Netherlands, *Journal of the American College of Cardiology*, **14**, 1609–15.
14. The TIMI Study Group (1989) Comparison of invasive and conservative strategies after treatment with intravenous tissue plasminogen activator in acute myocardial infarction: Results of the Thrombolysis in Myocardial Infarction (TIMI) Phase II Trial, *New England Journal of Medicine*, **320**, 618–27.
15. The SWIFT (Should We Intervene Following Thrombolysis) Trial Study Group (1991) The SWIFT trial of delayed elective intervention versus

conservative treatment after thrombolysis with anistreplase in acute myocardial infarction, *British Medical Journal*, **302**, 555–60.

16. Yusuf, S., Zucker, D., Peduzzi, P. Fisher, L.D., Takaro, T., Kennedy, J.W., Davis, K., *et al.* (1994) Effect of coronary bypass graft surgery on survival: overview of 10-years' results from randomised trials by the Coronary Artery Bypass Graft Surgery Trialists Collaboration. *Lancet*, **344**, 563–70.

17. Schulman, S.P., Achuff, S.C., Griffith, L.S., Humphries, J.O., Taylor, G.J., Mellits, E.D., Kennedy, M., *et al.* (1988) Prognostic cardiac catheterization variables in survivors of acute myocardial infarction: a five-year prospective study, *Journal of the American College of Cardiology*, **11**, 1164–72.

18. CASS Principal investigators and their associates (1983) Coronary Artery Surgery Study (CASS): a randomized trial of coronary artery bypass surgery: Survival data, *Circulation*, **68**, 939–50.

19. Whitford, D.L. and Southern, A.J. (1994) Audit of secondary prophylaxis after myocardial infarction, *British Medical Journal*, **309**, 1268–9.

20. Kottke, T.E., Battista, R.N., De Friese, G.H. and Brekke, M.L. (1988) Attributes of successful smoking cessation interventions in medical practice: A meta-analysis of 39 controlled trials. *Journal of the American Medical Association*, **259**, 2883–9.

21. Aberg, A., Bergstrand, R., Johansson, S., Ulvenstam, G., Vedin, A., Wedel, H., Wilhelmsson, C. and Wilhelmsen, L. (1983) Cessation of smoking after myocardial infarction: Effects on mortality after 10 years, *British Heart Journal*, **49**, 416–22.

22. Schuler, G., Hambrecht, R., Schlierf, G., Grunze, M., Methfessel, S., Hauer, K. and Kubler, W. (1992) Myocardial perfusion and regression of coronary artery disease in patients on a regimen of intensive physical exercise and low fat diet, *Journal of the American College of Cardiology*, **19**, 34–42.

23. Heath, G.W., Ehsani, A.A., Hagberg, J.M., Hinderliter, J.M. and Goldberg, A.P. (1983) Exercise training improves lipoprotein lipid profiles in patients with coronary artery disease, *American Heart Journal*, **105**, 889–95.

24. Meade, T.W., Ruddock, V., Stirling, Y., Chakrabarti, R. and Miller, G.J. (1993) Fibrinolytic activity, clotting factors, and long term incidence of ischaemic heart disease in the Northwick Park Heart Study, *Lancet*, **342**, 1076–9.

25. Ferguson, E., Bernier, L.L., Banta, G.R., Yu-Yahiro, J. and Schoomaker, E.B. (1987) Effects of exercise and conditioning on clotting and fibrinolytic activity in men, *Journal of Applied Physiology*, **62**, 1416–21.

26. The Scandinavian Simvastatin Survival Study Group (1994) Randomised trial of cholesterol lowering in 4444 patients with coronary heart disease: the Scandinavian Simvastatin Survival Study (4S), *Lancet*, **344**, 1383–9.

27. Collins, R., Peto, R., MacMahon, S., Hebert, D., Fiebach, N.H., Eberlein, K.A., Qizilbash, N., Taylor, J.O. and Hennekens, C.H. (1990) Effects of short-term reductions in diastolic blood pressure on stroke and coronary heart disease: evidence from an overview of randomised drug trials

considered in the context of observational epidemiology, *Lancet*, **335**, 827–38.

28. SHEP Co-operative Research Group (1991) Prevention of stroke by anti-hypertensive drug treatment in older persons with isolated systolic hypertension. Final results of the systolic hypertension in the elderly programme (SHEP), *Journal of the American Medical Association*, **265**, 3255–64.

29. Dahlof, B., Lindholm, L.H., Hansson, L., Schersten, B. and Ekhom, T. (1991) Morbidity and mortality in the Swedish Trial in Old Patients with Hypertension (STOP-Hypertension), *Lancet*, **338**, 1281–4.

30. Medical Research Council Working Party (1992) Medical Research Council trial of treatment of hypertension in older adults: principal results, *British Medical Journal*, **304**, 405–12.

31. Bundy, C., Carroll, D. Wallace, L. and Nagle, R. (1994) Psychological treatment of chronic stable angina pectoris, *Psychology and Health*, **10**, 69–77.

32. Todd, I.C. and Ballantyne, D. (1990) Antianginal efficacy of exercise training: a comparison with beta blockade, *British Heart Journal*, 64, 14–9.

33. Echt, D.S., Liebson, P.R., Mitchell, L.B., Peters, R.W., Obias-Manno, D., Barker, A.H. *et al.* (1991) Cardiac Arrhythmia Suppression Trial (CAST): mortality and morbidity in patients receiving encainide, flecainide or placebo, *New England Journal of Medicine*, **324**, 781–8.

34. Sullivan, M.J., Higginbotham, M.B. and Cobb, F.R. (1989) Exercise training in patients with chronic heart failure delays ventilatory anaerobic threshold and improves submaximal exercise performance, *Circulation*, **79**, 324–9.

35. Coats, A.J.S., Adamopoulos, S., Radaelli, A., McCance, A., Meyer, T.E., Bernardi, L., Solda, P.L., Davey, P., Ormerod, O., Forfar, C., Conway, J. and Sleight, P. (1992) Controlled trial of physical training in chronic heart failure: exercise performance, hemodynamics, ventilation and autonomic function, *Circulation*, **85**, 2119–31.

36. Coats, A.J.S. (1993) Exercise rehabilitation in chronic heart failure, *Journal of the American College of Cardiology*, **22 (suppl A)**, 172A–177A.

Further reading

American Heart Association (1994) Cardiac rehabilitation programs. A statement for health care professional, *Circulation*, **90**, 1602–10.

Haskell, W.L., Alderman, E.L., Fair, J.M., Maron, D.J., Mackey, S.E., Superko, H.R., Williams, P.T., Johnstone, I.M., Champagne, M.A., Krauss, R.M. and Farquhar, J.W. (1994) Effects of intensive multiple risk factor reduction on coronary atherosclerosis and clinical cardiac events in men and women with coronary artery disease, *Circulation*, **89**, 975–90.

Houston Miller, N., Taylor, C.B., Davidson, D.M., Hill, M.N. and Krantz, D.S. (1990) The efficacy of risk factor intervention and psychosocial aspects of cardiac rehabilitation. Position paper of the American Association of Cardiovascular and Pulmonary Rehabilitation, *Journal of Cardiopulmonary Rehabilitation*, **19**, 198–209.

Pyorola, K., DeBacker, G., Graham, I., Poole-Wilson, L. and Wood, D. (1994) Prevention of coronary heart disease in clinical practice. Recommendations of the Task Force of the European Society of Cardiology, European Atherosclerosis Society and European Society of Hypertension, *European Heart Journal*, **15**, 1300–31.

Chapter 4

Exercise Testing and Prescription

Summary

Exercise testing has a variety of uses in the management of patients with coronary heart disease, and also in other related conditions. The first section of this chapter reviews the uses, selection and interpretation of exercise tests; the second section discusses the prescription and evaluation of exercise as a therapeutic modality, and the structure of exercise sessions in a cardiac rehabilitation setting.

SECTION 1: MAJOR APPLICATIONS OF EXERCISE TESTING

The following are the major applications of exercise in the cardiology setting:

- Diagnostic:
    Identification of patient with CHD;
    Severity of CHD;
    Establishing cause of symptoms.
- Prognostic:
    Identification of high- moderate- and low-risk patients;
    Identification of patients who will benefit from intervention.
- Evaluation of therapy:
    Effectiveness of the selected intervention.
- Determination of functional capacity:
    Degree of incapacity and cause;
    Determination of safe exercise intensities for exercise prescription.
- Specific uses:
    Evaluation of exercise blood pressure, heart rate, or ventilatory responses;
    Detection of exercise-induced events, e.g. arrhythmias, left ventricular function, oxygen desaturation, etc.

Exercise tests

Formal or informal

Informal exercise tests, much used in practice, assess the ability of a patient to perform simple daily tasks or walking by simple observation – perhaps with measurement of the speed of task completion, combined with simple physiological monitoring, such as heart rate or respiratory rate. This approach is useful in estimating a patient's capacity quickly and inexpensively, but the information obtainable is limited and there is little standardization of test procedures. Numerous formal exercise protocols exist, utilizing a variety of different exercise modes which are discussed in detail later. Selection depends on the test objective(s); if the purpose is diagnostic or prognostic then a progressive, incremental test to maximal or symptom-limited effort is indicated; this is also the case if functional capacity is to be determined as a basis for exercise prescription. If the priority is to measure physiological responses to standard exercise (to detect exercise-induced events or to monitor improvements in fitness) then a constant load test may be required. Whatever the purpose, standardization of the test is crucial; unless this is rigorously maintained, the value of repeated testing of one patient is greatly reduced and inter-individual comparisions are ill-founded. Ways in which standardization is ensured are discussed later in this chapter. During the last 20 years greater knowledge concerning indications for testing, contra-indications, and end-points have combined to increase the safety of exercise testing as a procedure[1,2].

Diagnosis: sensitivity and specificity

The reliability of any diagnostic test depends on the sensitivity and specificity of the test. 'Sensitivity' and 'specificity' arc the terms used to define how effectively a test distinguishes between individuals with and without disease. 'Sensitivity' refers to the percentage of times that the test elicits an abnormal result when a diseased individual is tested (a true-positive test) whereas 'specificity' is the percentage of times that the test elicits a normal result when a disease-free individual is tested (a true-negative test).

The sensitivity of exercise electrocardiogram (ECG) testing in detecting CHD is increased by the use of maximal protocols, multiple lead monitoring and the adoption of additional criteria (such as poor blood pressure response and low exercise capacity) to determine an abnormal test result. However, there is an inverse relationship between sensitivity and specificity which means that greater sensitivity (the ability to identify diseased individuals) is usually achieved at the cost of decreased specificity (the ability to identify those without disease) and vice-versa. For example, if the criterion for an abnormal test is altered from 1 mm ST-segment depression to 2 mm, the percentage of people without disease who have a normal test result will increase (improved specificity). However, diseased individuals who exhibit ST-segment depression less than 2 mm will not be distinguished from those without disease and consequently the percentage of true-positives (the sensitivity of the test) will have been reduced. The major problem with using exercise testing for the detection of CHD is its relatively low sensitivity. For instance in asymptomatic men, exercise testing results in an average sensitivity of 61% which renders it impractical as a routine screening procedure. In women, exercise testing is (for reasons not fully understood) less sensitive and specific than in men. The concept of relative risk or predictive value is, therefore, central to understanding the diagnostic capabilities of exercise testing.

Diagnosis: predictive value

The accuracy with which a test result identifies diseased or non-diseased individuals is referred to as the predictive value of the test. In other words, the predictive value is the probability that a positive test represents disease in an individual and a negative test represents absence of disease. The major determinant of predictive value is directly related to the prevalence of disease within the population to which the individual belongs. If, for instance, on the basis of known risk factors such as increasing age, male gender and history of angina, the pre-test likelihood of disease in a given individual is low, an abnormal test is likely to be a false-positive. An abnormal result in an individual with a strong pre-test likelihood of disease will, in contrast, have a high predictive value. As a consequence, exercise testing is of greatest diagnostic use when the pre-test likelihood of CHD is equivocal; for instance a 55-year-old man with atypical angina has approximately a 50–60% likelihood of having CHD before testing is carried out. Following an exercise ECG, the likelihood is increased to 90% if the test proves positive and reduced to 30% if negative. Figure 4.1 provides a range of predictive values for exercise tests based on the prevalence of CHD in various sub-groups of individuals, and the cut-off level of diagnostic ST-segment level depression. The likelihood of disease may be further defined by additional information about smoking, blood pressure, serum cholesterol levels and family history of CHD.

Diagnosis: imaging during exercise testing

The predictive value of exercise testing can be improved by the addition of newer imaging modalities which can support the ECG changes in correctly identifying myocardial ischaemia. Advances in the radionuclide methods such as thallium scintigraphy can assess areas of reversible thallium uptake highly suggestive of reversible myocardial perfusion defects. Sensitivity and specificity rates have been reported to be 10–15% greater when radionuclide imaging is employed compared to standard exercise ECG tests alone. Other imaging techniques which can estimate blood flow include positron emission tomography (PET) scanning, or ultra-fast computed X-ray tomography with contrast injection. These remain expensive and are available only in selected research settings at present.

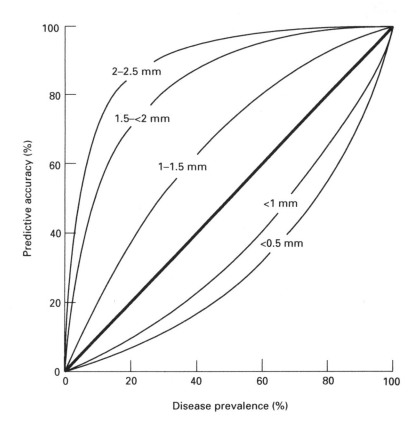

Figure 4.1 Family of S-T segment depression curves (Reproduced with permission from the *American Journal of Cardiology*.)

Sensitivity and specificity can also be increased by assessing the functional consequences of impaired myocardial blood flow rather than imaging the flow itself. Regional ventricular wall motion is impaired in the area subserved by a stenosed coronary artery. This can be detected by echocardiography, magnetic resonance imaging or radionuclide ventriculography if performed during exercise stress. Whilst there are technical difficulties with these methods, they can lead to an increase in precision in detecting functionally important CHD.

Lastly, the mode of stress can be altered to improve exercise testing applicability and precision. In patients unable to exercise for non-cardiac reasons, alternative cardiac stress tests can be used, combined with symptoms, ECG or any of the imaging modes mentioned above. These stresses include dobutamine, a β- and dopamine-receptor agonist which mimics many of the cardiovascular effects of exercise, or dipyridamole or adenosine which lead to blood flow diversion away from a stenosed artery due to selective vasodilatation of non-stenosed arteries.

Prognosis

Numerous investigators have demonstrated that responses to exercise testing soon after myocardial infarction (MI) or in established CHD or heart failure can enable predictions to be made about the severity of the disease and its probable course, i.e. the prognosis. Risk stratification identifies sub-groups of patients who may be at high risk for future clinical episodes and allows further diagnostic evaluation and medical and surgical intervention to be directed at those who will derive the greatest benefit. In addition, exercise testing distinguishes those at low risk who require less intensive evaluation and treatment and who are candidates for early rehabilitation and resumption of customary physical activities and work.

Overall mortality during the first year following acute MI is approximately 10%. More than half of these deaths occur within the first three months. First year re-infarction and the development of unstable angina pectoris are also concentrated in the early post-infarction period. The three main independent predictors of morbidity and mortality in post-MI patients are: left ventricular (LV) dysfunction, the amount of myocardium in jeopardy from ischaemia, and the propensity to ventricular arrhythmias. Both early, low level pre-discharge exercise testing and symptom-limited testing 3–4 weeks post-infarct have been found to be clinically predictive of risk of future events. Risk stratification is, however, based on patient populations and can only provide guidelines for likely outcomes in individual patients.

Exercise testing elicits a variety of electrocardiographic, haemodynamic and symptomatic responses. The question of which variables, either independently or in concert with others, are predictive of poor prognosis is complex and beyond the scope of this chapter. Those responses recognized as being of highest prognostic significance have been summarized but for more detailed coverage the reader is referred to several reviews of this topic[2-4].

In the absence of limiting orthopaedic, pulmonary or peripheral vascular disease, an exercise capacity less than 4 metabolic equivalents (METS) (one MET is the resting metabolic rate and equivalent to an oxygen uptake of 3.5 ml/kg/min) reflects severe left ventricular dysfunction and is indicative of a poor prognosis. Failure of systolic blood pressure to rise above the resting value during exercise or exercise-induced hypotension also suggests left ventricular dysfunction or severe myocardial ischaemia and hence a poor prognosis. Poor blood pressure response and low exercise capacity, although often associated, have independent prognostic significance.

The prognostic significance of ischaemic ST-segment changes depends upon their magnitude and the heart rate at which they become apparent. Generally, the lower the work load at which changes occur, the poorer is the prognosis. Changes which occur at higher workloads do not have the same significance, i.e. survival in patients with positive tests appears to be highly related to exercise capacity. The Coronary Artery Surgery Study (CASS) reported that the benefit of coronary bypass surgery was greatest in those patients who showed 1 mm ST-segment depression at work loads less than 5 METS[5]. In contrast, no benefit was seen in those patients who were able to exceed 10 METS. Premature ventricular complexes elicited during exercise are associated with greater risk of subsequent cardiac events but are less sensitive prognostically than low work capacity, ischaemic abnormalities or blood pressure responses.

Despite the contribution of exercise testing in assessing prognosis, the importance of good clinical judgement should be underlined. In a meta-analysis of studies which attempted to identify the test responses most predictive of poor prognosis, patients considered eligible for testing were found to constitute a relatively low-risk group compared with those who did not fulfil the eligibility criteria[3].

Evaluation of therapy

Exercise testing may be used to evaluate pharmacological management and the efficacy of medical or surgical interventions and exercise prescription within CR programmes. The most useful information is yielded when testing is performed before and after the intervention, for instance percutaneous transluminal coronary angioplasty (PTCA) or coronary artery bypass graft (CABG) surgery. In the case of evaluating the effectiveness of various agents in controlling exercise-induced angina, arrhythmias or hypertension, serial exercise testing may be indicated in order to optimize therapy.

Determination of functional capacity

The objective of determining functional capacity is to assess the maximal exercise intensity which an individual can perform without the appearance of symptoms or measurable detrimental variables such as ST-segment depression, hypotension or arrhythmias. On the basis of the test result, decisions can be made about the safety of the patient to perform tasks of everyday living, resume recreational activities and meet occupational requirements. Specifically, the functional capacity of the patient, in METS, can be compared with the MET values (metabolic 'cost', energy requirements) of the most common activities of daily living (Table 4.1); decisions about his or her capability to live independently or resume work can be made with more objectivity. In some cases specialist testing which simulates the demands of specific occupations may be appropriate.

Periodic re-assessment of functional capacity in patients enrolled in supervised rehabilitation programmes is also helpful, not only to quantify the effectiveness of the intervention but also to ensure that, as functional capacity increases in response to training, prescribed exercise levels are adjusted in order to maintain the training stimulus. Evaluation of participants' individual progression or regression is covered in more detail later in this chapter.

Exercise testing which determines functional capacity has proved to be therapeutic in its own right. Patients are apparently reassured by their ability to

Table 4.1 Energy requirements in METS (multiples of resting rate, oxygen uptake equivalent of 1 MET is 3.5 ml/kg/min) of activities of daily living. (Reprinted with permission from Ainsworth *et al.* (1993)[6].)

Activity	MET value
Personal care	
Bathing	2.0
Dressing/undressing	2.5
Showering	4.0
Cleaning	
Light, e.g. dusting, vacuuming, changing beds	2.5
Heavy, major, e.g. washing windows, mopping	4.5
Moving furniture	6.0
Sweeping garage	4.0
Light domestic activities	
Washing up, serving food, putting away groceries	2.5
Ironing	2.3
DIY activities	
Carpentry	3.01–6.0
Laying carpets/linoleum	4.5
Decorating	4.5
Wiring/plumbing	3.0
Food shopping	
Using trolley	3.5
Walking, standing shopping	2.0–2.3
Gardening	
Digging	5.0
Mowing lawn (powered hand mower)	4.5
Raking	4.0
Shovelling snow	6.0

complete the test without incident and this may lead to increased activity at home and greater compliance with the prescribed exercise regimen. It has been reported that pre-discharge testing is independently associated with lower mortality and reduced incidence of subsequent clinical events[4].

An exercise test is a prerequisite for individual exercise prescription. Measurement of peak oxygen uptake, heart rate, blood pressure, rating of perceived exertion (RPE), ECG and symptoms form the objective basis on which the prescription is developed. Perhaps the most fundamental of these is the maximal oxygen uptake (VO_{2max}) as this is the main determinant of the level of sundry responses to exercise; metabolic, cardiovascular, hormonal and thermoregulatory responses are all dictated by the percentage of the individual's VO_{2max} that a particular exercise level represents. Exercise of a given absolute exercise intensity may represent 50% VO_{2max} for one patient but maybe 80% for another, with correspondingly different responses. If the level of physiological stress, and therefore the adaptive potential, is to be at a desirable level for each individual, it is vital that assessment of functional capacity is made.

Exercise testing procedures

Choice of protocols

As mentioned above, the selection of a suitable protocol depends on the objectives of the test. Incremental tests, where exercise intensity is increased progressively to exhaustion, either fatigue- or symptom-limited, are used both as a diagnostic tool and to determine functional capacity. This is traditionally measured as the VO_{2max} because of the linear relationship between oxygen uptake and exercise intensity (measured as work rate on a cycle ergometer or combination of speed and grade on a treadmill). In patients with CHD, it is influenced by disease severity as well as by genetic predisposition and habitual physical activity level – the factors which influence VO_{2max} in healthy individuals. For this reason the term VO_{2peak} is often preferred for this patient group and will be used hereafter in relation to the maximal value which can be attained in patients with CHD. (Some of the protocols most widely employed to determine this quantity are discussed subsequently.)

Cycle ergometer protocols should begin with an 'unloaded' stage, followed by progressive increments of between 25 and 50 watts, every 2 to 3 minutes. On isokinetic ergometers work rate is independent of pedal frequency. On other types of ergometer, the popular and robust Monarks for example, this is not the case and pedalling cadence must be controlled if the test is to be standardized. Work rate is best varied by increasing the resistive force, whilst maintaining a constant pedal frequency; 50 rpm is comfortable for most patients. (See Table 4.2)

Whether the levels of an incremental exercise test should increase in a stepwise manner or continuously depends on the purpose of the test; if it is for measurement of the physiological responses to exercise then longer stages allow steady-state conditions to develop – but stages must be at least 4 minutes long to achieve

Table 4.2 Energy expenditure during cycle ergometry. Source of data: Action Heart, Dudley.

Work rate		Oxygen uptake			
				METS	
Watts	kgm.min^{-1}	litres.min^{-1}	60 kg	75 kg	100 kg
50	300	0.9	4.3	3.4	2.6
100	600	1.5	7.1	5.7	4.3
150	900	2.1	10.0	8.0	6.0
200	1200	2.8	13.3	10.7	8.0
250	1500	3.5	16.7	13.3	10.0
300	1800	4.2	20.0	16.0	12.0

Table 4.3 Commonly used treadmill protocols with MET values for each stage or minute interval completed.

Bruce protocol

Stage	Speed (mph)	Grade (%)	Stage length (min)	MET value
1	1.7	10	3	5
2	2.5	12	3	7
3	3.4	14	3	9
4	4.2	16	3	11
5	5.0	18	3	13

Modified Bruce (Sheffield)

Stage	Speed (mph)	Grade (%)	Stage length (min)	MET value
1	1.7	0	3	2.3
2	1.7	5	3	3.5
3	1.7	10	3	4.8
4	2.5	12	3	6.6
5	3.4	14	3	8.4
6	4.2	16	3	10.2

Balke

Stage	Speed (mph)	Grade (%)	Stage length (min)	MET value
1	3	0	3	3
2	3	2	3	4
3	3	5	3	5
4	3	7.5	3	6
5	3	10	3	7
6	3	12.5	3	8

this, longer than the stages in any of the commonly used protocols in Table 4.3; if the test function is purely to evaluate functional capacity then either short stages or a continuous increase in intensity is preferable. Excessively long tests should be avoided because they are poorly reproducible and because local muscle fatigue may cause the test to be ended prematurely before VO_{2peak} is attained.

There is, of course, an interaction between test duration and the size of the increment employed: too steep an increase in load in incremental tests means inadequate time for proper physiological monitoring, poor test sensitivity and that the test is poorly tolerated by the patient. Although it is unlikely that there is a single protocol ideally suited to all the uses of exercise testing, it does appear that a progressive test lasting about 12 minutes is close to optimal for evaluation of VO_{2peak}.

Endurance tests

Although maximal exercise performance, dictated by VO_{2peak} is important, the more important physiological goal for the patient is endurance (stamina). This is best defined as the ability to sustain exercise which represents a high proportion of personal VO_{2peak} and contributes greatly to a patient's capability for the exercise demands of everyday life. It is independent of VO_{2peak}; someone whose functional capacity is constrained by disease or by genetic predisposition can still develop good endurance becaues this characteristic depends largely on the metabolic 'quality' of the muscles.

Endurance is ideally measured as the maximal time for which an individual can maintain exercise at, say, 60–70% of previously determined VO_{2peak}. The choice of too low an exercise intensity (relative to VO_{2peak}) can lead to excessively long tests which are poorly reproducible, perhaps because boredom contributes to the reasons for termination. If it is not desired to measure endurance directly, i.e. to exercise the patient to fatigue, an alternative is to examine the changes over time in the physiological responses to this level of exercise (for example, ventilation, heart rate and blood lactate concentration). This will give an indication of whether the patient could *sustain* the exercise; if a 'steady state' is evident the exercise is probably sustainable, if progressive increases in these responses are evident over, say, 5 to 10 minutes then endurance would be poor. Endurance tests allow objective monitoring of physiological responses to a constant sub-maximal work load, comparable to many of the activities of daily living, but to be worthwhile require prior assessment of functional capacity.

Mode of exercise

Although individual muscle groups can be tested for strength and resistance to fatigue, the relevant exercise tests for the majority of CHD patients are those which demand a sustained high cardiac output, i.e. dynamic exercise with the body's large muscle groups. Theoretically, walking, swimming, running, rowing, cycling or stepping would all be suitable but in practice treadmill walking test and stationary cycling are the two most popular. The choice depends on local factors, including cost and space.

A treadmill test achieves the greater cardiovascular challenge because it involves a larger muscle mass and is possibly therefore the preferred mode. Moreover, not all patients are familiar with cycling and many find it difficult to maintain a steady cadence, so that test standardization is poor with many ergometers. On the other hand, there may be greater security for patients with cycle ergometry: they are seated and can stop with safety at any time. Treadmill walking is vastly different from free walking and patients may feel unstable and that they have less control over the test. The use of hand rails diminishes these problems but of course decreases the work done and therefore the oxygen uptake; this leads to over-estimation of capacity and to loss of standardization. External work rate can be determined on a cycle ergometer, whereas in treadmill testing this depends on the weight of the subject. A fundamental issue is that during cycle ergometry the body mass is supported. If one of the test's objectives is to describe the patient's level of exercise capacity in everyday life, then it may be important to test in a situation where the patient has to support his or her own body weight.

Peak heart rates during cycle ergometry are not usually very different from values obtained during treadmill exercise; however, VO_{2peak} is about 5–10% lower and systolic blood pressure tends to be somewhat higher, probably because of the isometric contractions of the arm muscles in gripping the handlebars. Blood lactate concentrations tend to be higher during exercise of a given proportion of VO_{2peak} during cycling than during treadmill exercise. Where neither a treadmill nor a cycle ergometer are available, externally-paced stepping or walking make perfectly acceptable alternatives with which a good level of standardization can be achieved. The same principles of testing apply: the test should be graded, with short or longer test stages according to objectives.

A new approach not yet examined fully in patients with CHD is the shuttle walking test where patients walk up and down a 10 metre course at a pace determined by an audio signal; the pace of walking increases each minute until the patient cannot cover the required distance in the time interval specified[7]. This protocol was developed for use with patients with chronic obstructive pulmonary disease but may prove more widely applicable; it would not, however, be suitable where ECG monitoring would be required. Tasks such as the distance which can be walked in a specified time, e.g. 6 or 12 minute walk tests, or the time taken to complete a set task, e.g. the corridor walk test, can also be useful; it is important to remember, however, that these measure exercise performance, which of course depends on *both* functional capacity and endurance.

Standardization

Whatever mode of exercise and protocol employed the need for standardization is self-evident; if this is poor then comparisions of test performance or physiological responses, either within or between patients, will be invalid. Calibration of the ergometer(s) is the starting point: both the belt speed and the inclination of a treadmill should be measured at regular intervals; mechanically-braked cycle ergometers are easy to calibrate but more problems will be encountered with electronically braked models which may have to be dealt with by the manu-facturer.

Another important contribution to good standardization comes from adequate patient familiarization to both the mode of exercise and any equipment to be used for expired air collection. Familiarization to treadmill walking should include experience of stopping, starting and of changes in grade and speed. Time spent doing this should be regarded as an investment to secure good data and even a few minutes prior to the test will be repaid by ensuring that the patient is as comfortable as possible with what is required.

Physiological monitoring

Heart rate and blood pressure

A variety of physiological responses can be measured during an exercise test. It is almost universal to monitor heart rate as an assessment of the level of cardio-vascular stress. Often, this can best be performed by continuous monitoring of the electrocardiogram. This, of course, has other advantages (see below). There are limitations to relying on heart rate as a measure of exercise intensity because maximal heart rates differ markedly between individuals. It may be advisable to gather additional information through ratings of perceived exertion (see below), particularly when patients are taking medication that restricts the heart rate response.

Blood pressure is usually also monitored as, in certain circumstances, an evaluation of peak exercise blood pressure can be useful; a fall in blood pressure during progressive exercise can be a marker of severe coronary artery disease. It should be recognized, however, that non-invasive monitoring of diastolic blood pressure is not reliable during exercise; even measurement of systolic blood pressure is less accurate than at rest.

Electrocardiography

Exercise electrocardiography using an incremental protocol is the most common and practical technique for evaluating cardiac perfusion and function. Although other non-invasive tests have proved more sensitive for the diagnosis of CHD, standard exercise ECG testing yields a large amount of clinically relevant infor-mation and is widely available, reliable and cost-effective. Consequently, it plays an increasingly significant role in the diagnosis, prognosis, treatment and reha-bilitation phases of CHD management. The interpretation of an exercise ECG test is not restricted to analysis of the ECG recording but takes in important information on heart rate, blood pressure and symptomatic responses to exercise. A test is considered positive if certain ECG changes (see below) occur on exercise, but in addition it is important to know if classical anginal pain, or other symp-toms occur either simultaneously or separately from these changes. The criteria for significant ECG changes on exercise are dependent on the prevalence of the disease (as shown in Figure 4.1) and are inevitably arbitrary. Masters' original criterion of 0.5 mm ST-segment depression is now considered too sensitive and with too high a false postive rate, so that horizontal or down-sloping ST-segment depression of 1 mm in relation to the preceding isoelectric PR-segment is a more common criterion. Even when the ST-segment is up-sloping it can be considered positive if the ST level 80 msec after the terminal deflection of the QRS-complex (the J point) is depressed 1 mm. An alternative with a higher specificity is the use of 2 mm as the cut-off level.

Ratings of perceived exertion

In assessing the response to exercise it can be useful to know the level of perception of effort or distress of the subject. This can be assessed as an 'all embracing' measure or separately for fatigue, dyspnoea or intensity of chest pain. A perceived exertion scale (see Tables 4.4 and 4.5) allows quantification of the subjective intensity of exercise[8,9]. Ratings on Borg's scale are reproducible measures of exertion and have strong relationships with objective measures of the level of 'physiological stress', most fundamentally the percentage of VO_{2peak} which the exercise elicits. Most individuals will use the scales appropriately from first exposure, rating 60 to 75% VO_{2peak} as 'somewhat hard' or 'hard' (RPE 13 to 16 on the 15 point scale), but a minority will tend to underestimate during light-

Table 4.4 Rating of perceived exertion (RPE) (Borg 1973)[8]: 15-point category scale.

6	
7	Very, very light
8	
9	Very light
10	
11	Fairly light
12	
13	Somewhat hard
14	
15	Hard
16	
17	Very hard
18	
19	Very, very hard
20	

Table 4.5 Rating of perceived exertion (RPE) (Borg 1982)[9]: 10-point category-ratio scale.

0	Nothing at all
0.5	Very, very weak (just noticeable)
1	Very weak
2	Weak (light)
3	Moderate
4	Somewhat strong
5	Strong (heavy)
6	
7	Very strong
8	
9	
10	Very, very strong (almost maximal)
•	Maximal

to-moderate exercise and will require two to three trials before reliable ratings are made. As with any rating scale, it is important to give patients standardized instructions to minimize variation within and between individuals. Valid ratings can only be achieved from inevitably anxious patients if staff create a reassuring and non-judgmental atmosphere.

Respiratory gas exchange and arterial blood gases

Monitoring respiratory gas exchange during exercise testing can give added information. It is more often used in the assessment of fitness and in the evaluation of patients with impaired left ventricular function or heart failure, than in the assessment of coronary artery disease *per se*. Several variables can be derived to assess the physiological response of the heart and lung to exercise. Maximal oxygen uptake is more objective and more reproducible than exercise duration, and has the advantage of being comparable at least partially between different modes and types of exercise test: evidence from healthy individuals suggests that values are on average some 8% higher when measured during treadmill walking or running than during cycling. In addition, the respiratory gas exchange ratio (RER) on peak exercise (ratio of rate of carbon dioxide production to oxygen uptake) can tell us something about the factors limiting exercise.

Where cardiac function and hence cardiac output is the limiting factor, there is an inadequate perfusion of the exercising muscle and hence the muscle increasingly relies on anaerobic glycolysis – producing an increase in carbon dioxide excretion and hence RER as lactic acid (the 'end product' of this series of reactions) is buffered by plasma bicarbonate. If this ratio remains below 1.0 then exercise has probably not been limited by cardiac output and alternative causes should be sought. This may be anginal chest pain without functional cardiac limitation, other unpleasant symptoms leading to exercise termination, or lung dysfunction. In the latter case some alteration in arterial blood gases is seen on exercise such as arterial oxygen desaturation or an increase in arterial carbon dioxide levels. These changes are very unusual in cardiac failure alone and, where seen, indicate important lung disease, pulmonary shunting of blood or ventilation/perfusion mismatching. The measurement of the ventilatory response to exercise can be useful in evaluating causes of dyspnoea, especially when combined with measurement of arterial blood gases. In psychogenic dyspnoea, generated by high levels of patient anxiety, there is hyperventilation leading to blowing off carbon dioxide and low arterial carbon dioxide levels, associated with termination of exercise due to dyspnoea in the absence of a high RER.

A methodological note is justified here: accuracy in measurement of oxygen and carbon dioxide in expired air is a prerequisite if RER values are to be meaningful. Artefactual values will also occur if the patient is unfamiliar with the equipment used to collect expired air.

Perfusion or functional imaging

Exercise testing can be combined with other imaging modalities such as thallium scintigraphy to assess myocardial perfusion, or echocardiography or magnetic resonance imaging to look at regional myocardial wall motion abnormalities. These can increase the diagnostic power of an exercise test by an independent assessment of the significance of the ECG changes seen. These tests are more expensive and, in the case of nuclear techniques, their use may be limited by access to appropriate facilities. They can, however, increase the specificity of the evaluation of cardiac ischaemia, and have an important role in selected cases.

Other, more detailed, forms of physiological monitoring can play a role in evaluating specific components of the exercise response, such as cardiac output, ventricular filling pressures or peripheral organ blood flow, but the discussion of these measurements is beyond the scope of this chapter.

End-points for test

In the early post-infarct period maximal exercise testing is not recommended. The pre-discharge test, usually performed at about 1 week after the myocardial infarction, should not exceed the second stage of the Bruce protocol in intensity (equivalent to 7 METS, or stage 5 of the Balke protocol). When testing is performed at least one month after the infarct symptom-limited tests can be performed. In these tests the patient is encouraged to exercise until his or her limit is reached. This may be because of the development of unpleasant chest pain, dyspnoea, muscular fatigue, or general exhaustion. These can be quantified by RPE scores, or independently assessed by the respiratory exchange ratio where respiratory gas exchange data are being acquired.

Exercise tests can also be terminated early when certain physiological end-points have been reached, such as reaching a predicted maximal heart rate (220 – age in years for males; 200 – age for females) or certain values of blood pressure (exceeding 250 systolic, or showing a progressive fall with increasing exercise load). The development of significant ECG changes, such as 2 mm ST-segment depression (see page 57) may lead to termination of the test if enough diagnostic information has been obtained (clearly positive result at low work-load), or if exaggerated ST-segment changes (greater than 4 mm depression, significant ST-elevation) have occurred. Runs of ventricular tachycardia, multifocal ventricular ectopics, and other significant arrhythmias should also lead to termination of the test.

Clinical medical indications and contraindications for exercise testing

Exercise testing is useful in assessing new presentations and also the treatment of angina, atypical chest pains, post-myocardial infarction, and left ventricular dysfunction and heart failure. In addition, it has a limited role in screening high risk individuals. If the population screened has a low prevalence of CHD, however, the problems of false positive tests should not be forgotten. Other specific cases, such as exercise-induced hypertension or hypotension, exercise-induced arrhythmias or assessment of unusual symptoms may be indications for exercise testing.

Certain medical conditions increase the risk of exercise testing and should be considered relative or absolute contraindications to maximal exercise testing. These include:

- Acute febrile illness
- Viral infections
- Severe uncontrolled hypertension

} Absolute contraindications

- Hypertrophic cardiomyopathy
- Aortic stenosis
- Significant arrhythmias

} Relative contraindications

Other medical conditions affecting exercise testing, procedures or interpretation

The results of exercise testing can be affected by the medical condition of the patient. For example in the presence of bundle branch block on the resting ECG, or exercise-induced bundle branch block, conventional ST-segment criteria for assessing a positive result are unreliable and cannot be utilized. In the presence of left ventricular hypertrophy with resting repolarization changes, such as in hypertension, then it may be difficult to interpret further changes in the ST-segment with exercise. ST-segment changes in this circumstance need not necessarily indicate myocardial ischaemia. Similarly ST/T-wave changes can be produced by digoxin, and where present can give false-positive changes on exercise testing. In this situation, where exercise testing alone may be unreliable, perfusion imaging (as discussed earlier) may be of use in addition to an exercise test.

Patients with conditions leading to exercise intolerance such as lung disorders, orthopaedic or peripheral vascular disorders or neurological disorders may be unable to perform sufficient exercise to stress the heart adequately to detect myocardial ischaemia. In these cases alternative stress agents such as adenosine, dipyridamole or dobutamine may be used (see above).

Effect of cardiovascular and other drugs on the design and interpretation of tests

Certain drugs can affect either exercise performance or the response of the heart to exercise. The effect of digoxin on the ST-segment has been mentioned above. Beta-blockers, some calcium antagonists and to a lesser extent, angiotensin-inhibiting enzymes (ACE inhibitors) slow the heart rate, and have an anti-ischaemic effect. For both these reasons patients are less likely to demonstrate an ischaemic ECG response to exercise. This is a disadvantage if the exercise test is being used to diagnose CHD in cases where high sensitivity is required. As a result, it is commonly recommended to withdraw beta-blockers for several drug half-lives before exercise testing. If, however, the exercise ECG is being used to assess the functional capacity or ischaemic threshold of a patient with known CHD, then his/her status on optimal therapy is more useful; such patients should be studied on their usual medication which would frequently include beta-blockers.

Nitrates dilate the coronary arteries and reduce the loading conditions of the heart – both of which exert an anti-anginal and anti-ischaemic effect. When active this would lessen the sensitivity of the test in detecting structural CHD, but increase the relevance of the test result to the status of the treated patient. Similar considerations pertain to other anti-anginal drug groups, including the calcium antagonists. Some drugs increase heart rate and may lead to coronary vasoconstriction – such as the sympathomimetics, infrequently used on a regular basis but sometimes found in cough and cold remedies. These may exaggerate a positive exercise ECG. Anti-hypertensive agents should generally be taken on the day of the test to prevent an exaggerated hypertensive response, although a drug-free period of 4 hours prior to exercise testing is recommended. Similarly regular bronchodilators should be taken.

SECTION II – EXERCISE PRESCRIPTION

Indications and contraindications to exercise prescription

Exercise training should be considered part of the routine management of stable patients with the following cardiovascular conditions[10]:

- Angina
- Post-myocardial infarction
- Left ventricular dysfunction
- Heart failure, hypertension
- Hyperlipidaemia.

It is also useful in the management of related and overlapping conditions, including:

- Obesity
- Diabetes
- Chronic renal failure
- Chronic lung disease
- Peripheral vascular disease.

By contrast, the list of contraindications is relatively short, and it predominantly includes patients with unstable symptoms or conditions. In addition, exercise should not be encouraged in:

- Hypertrophic obstructive cardiomyopathy;
- Significant aortic stenosis;
- Acute febrile illness;
- Viral infection;
- Active myocarditis;
- Exercise-induced ventricular arrhythmias (see pp. 48, 88).

Effect of non-cardiac disease on exercise prescription

Non-cardiac disease can affect exercise prescription by: interfering with the ability of the patients to perform the exercise, by being a contraindication to training, or by blocking the training effects. Where a patient is able to walk for more than 10 minutes at a moderate pace there is the possibility of useful training effects. Even in patients more severely limited, useful training can occur by the use of single-limb or limited range-of-muscle-group exercise. These can be performed sequentially to enable a diverse training stimulus while not over-stressing the cardiopulmonary system at any one time. A list of conditions that have shown improvement with training have been mentioned above; in contrast there are few in which training is impossible. These include:

- Large strokes;
- Severe arthritis;
- Orthopaedic disability;
- Neuropathies;
- Severe neuromuscular disorders.

In asthma, exercise may provoke bronchospasm and hence make training difficult, but if this can be avoided by prior bronchodilator therapy, the effects of training on lung and respiratory muscle function are likely to prove beneficial. The authors are not aware of any condition that specifically prevents a cardiovascular, or muscular training effect. The benefits of training are both profound and extensive[11], and should be made available to as wide a patient population as possible.

Interaction between medication and exercise prescription

Little is known of the interaction between pharmacological agents and training effects. Beta-blockers can increase fatigue and reduce the training stimulus of a bout of exercise but they do not preclude a training effect and, in the case of hypertension, the effects can be additive. Other agents which improve exercise tolerance may allow exercise training to be performed at a more beneficial level.

Exercise rehabilitation goals

The primary aims of exercise rehabilitation are to:

- Counteract the deleterious effects of bedrest;
- Avoid the deconditioning effects of inactivity imposed by disease;
- Improve responses to sub-maximal exercise bouts of daily life;
- Modify risk factors.

Consequences of inactivity

The consequences of inactivity are multifarious and rapid and are described for the healthy population; muscle fibre hypotrophy leads to a diminution of muscle mass and strength, and muscle oxidative capacity falls, reducing endurance. Marked decreases in whole body functional capacity are evident; classic studies in the late sixties showed a drop in VO_{2max} of 27% after three weeks of bed rest but even cessation of training whilst maintaining the normal activities of daily living results in a measurable decrease after 4–6 weeks. In patients with CHD the deleterious effects of bedrest also include moderate tachycardia (increasing cardiac work), orthostatic hypotension and increased risk of thromboembolism.

In older patients, inactivity-related decreases in functional capacities (of muscle groups or the whole body) are critically important. If VO_{2peak} has fallen below thresholds needed for tasks such as crossing a road safely, climbing stairs or rising from a low armless chair or toilet, then there are deleterious consequences for quality of life and individuals previously capable of living independently may no longer be able to do so.

Effects of exercise training in healthy people

Exercise 'training' may be defined as maintaining a regular programme of increased activity at levels greater than those usually performed. Just as inactivity decreases functional capacity, increased levels of exercise will stimulate beneficial adaptations as 'fitness' improves. In healthy people VO_{2max} can be increased with training by 6–30%, depending on the training regimen and the initial level of fitness (improvements are positively related to training intensity and inversely related to fitness level).

Maximal oxygen uptake is limited by a central component (cardiac output) and peripheral factors – in particular the capacity of skeletal muscle to extract oxygen from the blood. The most important change provoked by exercise training appears to be an increase in maximal cardiac output which arises from increased maximal stroke volume (maximal heart rates are unchanged).

Endurance is improved by two mechanisms:

First, a given bout of exercise constitutes a smaller percentage of the new, increased VO_{2max} and therefore the exercise provokes relatively less physiological 'stress' than before (for example, heart rate will be lower and plasma catecholamine concentrations and systolic blood pressure will be lower at the given level of exercise[12]); second, peripheral changes in the trained muscle profoundly enhance its oxidative capacity; activities of oxidative enzymes are increased (because of an increase in mitochondrial protein) and the microcirculation is improved. Both mean a greater capacity of oxidative adenosine triphosphate (ATP) re-synthesis with a correspondingly decreased reliance on glycolysis during standardized exercise and a consequent delay in the onset of fatigue.

The magnitude of the potential for local skeletal muscle adaptation should be emphasized; the VO_{2max} of athletes may be twice that of sedentary controls but the activity of mitochondrial enzymes is 3- to 4-fold higher. The stimulus appears to be a high chronic demand for oxygen consumption by the muscle; changes in oxidative capacity are therefore restricted to the muscles which are trained, as shown by studies in which only one leg is trained and enzyme activities in the untrained leg remain unchanged.

Effects of exercise training in cardiac patients

With rehabilitation, reported increases in VO_{2peak} are between 10% and 55% in MI patients and between 15% and 65% in coronary artery bypass graft (CABG) patients after three to six months of exercise training. These improvements are far greater than those seen for sedentary (but healthy) people who begin training, because of the contribution of the natural process of recovery. Activity-related increases appear to be due to peripheral adaptations of the muscles which have been trained (rather than changes in central circulatory capacity) resulting in an increase in oxygen extraction and utilization by skeletal muscle during exercise.

In selected CHD patients, however, it has been shown that high intensity exercise training can provoke central cardiovascular adaptations – for example, increased maximal stroke volume – in a manner similar to that evident for healthy adults[13]. The intensity of the training regimen employed in this study (> 85% of VO_{2peak}) was, however, inappropriate for the majority of cardiac patients. Most patients will derive benefit from the local metabolic adaptations of skeletal muscle in response to regimens of moderate intensity; the important message is that the benefits conferred will be greatest when a large muscle mass is trained.

The principal advantages of exercise training in the CHD patient are in the improved responses to the repeated sub-maximal exercise bouts of everyday living – an indirect benefit from increased peak performance. As described above for healthy people, these include a lower heart rate and systolic blood pressure; for the patient, the decrease in myocardial oxygen demands is particularly important. Suggestions of possible increases in myocardial vascularity, enhanced dilating capacity of coronary arteries and decreased progression (or even regression) of coronary atherosclerotic lesions remain unproven.

As far as the safety of exercise training is concerned, evidence shows that the incidence for cardiac arrest is 8.9 per million patient hours. Of these arrests, 86% were successfully resuscitated, giving an incidence of death of 1.3 per million patient hours. This compares favourably with the estimated death rate for joggers at 2.5 per million person-hours of jogging[14].

Risk factor modification

Despite the primacy of the need for improved exercise capability, the role of exercise in risk factor modification should not be forgotten. Recently, the important contribution, for healthy people, of the 'acute' effects of each exercise bout has received more attention[15]; acute effects include a raised post-exercise metabolic rate, dynamic changes in lipoprotein metabolism leading to increased synthesis of HDL, improved insulin sensitivity and decreased blood pressure. These effects all relate to local changes in the previously exercised skeletal muscle. They are evident after even light to moderate exercise, showing that a general increase in physical activity (probably not sufficient to provoke a traditional training response) is likely to contribute to the patient's continued well-being.

Individualized exercise prescription

When developing an individual training regimen, several factors must be considered with regard to the exercise:

- Mode
- Intensity
- Frequency
- Duration
- Rate of progression
- Strength training.

Mode

On the basis of both the 'chronic' (adaptive) and 'acute' responses to exercise which have been considered above, endurance (aerobic) exercise should be the major component of the exercise regimen for CHD patients. Large increases in energy expenditure can be achieved because it can be sustained for some time without fatigue. Such exercise demands that a high cardiac output be maintained for a prolonged period. The dynamic use of large muscle groups causes local vasodilation and consequently there is a fall in peripheral resistance which opposes the rise in blood pressure otherwise associated with increased cardiac output, an important consideration for safety. Benefits – short-term and long-term – associated with peripheral changes localized to the exercised muscle will also be maximized when the muscle mass employed is large.

The inclusion of a variety of modes of exercise will minimize the incidence of over-use injuries, maximize peripheral adaptation (as for example when activities which require a contribution from both upper and lower body musculature are included) and will increase patient motivation. Nevertheless, walking should be the mainstay of rehabilitation – particularly in the early stages and when activity is unsupervised – either as part of home-based programmes or between supervised sessions.

Intensity

This issue is critical for risk-benefit assessment because vigorous activity carries a high risk of precipitating an MI[16]. Benefit in terms of a substantially lower risk of first coronary events in asymptomatic men is associated with moderate activity like walking and cycling[17], as well as more vigorous activity and it is plausible that this may also be the case for patients. A satisfactory training effect can result from exercise regimens of moderate intensity, compensated by longer duration and greater frequency[18]. Moreover, this approach appears to be associated with better adherence, is characterized by greater safety, can be undertaken with less professional supervision and is therefore less costly; it also fosters the important progressive transition to independence in exercising.

Intensity: prescribing and monitoring intensity of exercise

Intensity should, ideally, be related to the individual's previously determined VO_{2peak} because the proportion of VO_{2peak} represented by a particular bout of exercise dictates the level of the metabolic and physiological responses that will be elicited. The percentage of functional capacity that a given individual can sustain is quite variable but improves with endurance fitness. In general, exercise during conditioning sessions should be within the range 40–85% of functional capacity[2]. Typically, cardiac patients beginning an exercise programme will need to start at 40–60% of VO_{2peak}.

Different methods are available to prescribe and monitor exercise intensity to ensure an intensity that allows a reasonable period of exercise (say, 15–50 minutes) to be performed. All methods should all be regarded as a guide and modified according to the patient's response; the subject's previous levels of fitness and co-existing orthopaedic or other problems (e.g. being overweight) must be taken into account.

Intensity: use of heart rate

There are three different ways of using heart rate as a means of controlling intensity: (1) This requires the availability of a facility to establish the relationship between heart rate and oxygen uptake (up to VO_{2peak}) for an individual. The range of heart rates associated with the desired percentages of functional capacity can then be determined directly; (2) If the maximal heart rate is known but not VO_{2peak}, then the patient's heart rate range can be identified, i.e. the difference between maximal and resting heart rate; 60–80% of the heart rate range is known to be equivalent to 60–80% of VO_{2peak}. A problem here is the resting heart rate since this is affected by levels of anxiety; nevertheless it is convenient in that equivalent percentages of maximal heart rate and VO_{2peak} are numerically equal; (3) A simple approach is to use a fixed percentage of maximal heart rate. This relies on the observation that 70–85% of maximal heart rate is equivalent to about 60–80% of VO_{2peak} (the numerical difference is attributable to the fact that, as maximal effort is approached, oxygen uptake increases relatively less than heart rate). Heart rate monitoring may be achieved by telemetry of either ECG (for high-risk patients) or heart rate, or by pulse palpation. If patients are to employ the latter method themselves, careful instruction and sufficient practice are required.

There are circumstances when it is not practical to determine an individual's true maximal heart rate, and in these cases pre-decided age-adjusted maximal heart rates are used (220 – age in years for males; 200 – age for females). The standard deviation for maximal heart rate during exercise is, however, $\pm$ 10 beats per minute. Consequently, some individuals will have an actual maximum heart rate as much as 20 beats per minute higher or lower than that predicted. Predicted maximal heart rates should, therefore, only be used as a guide and other responses including RPE should be monitored.

Intensity: use of perceived exertion scales

Where heart rate cannot be used as the basis for prescription, e.g. because of the effects of medication, an alternative is the rating of perceived exertion (RPE) described earlier. Cardiorespiratory and metabolic variables are strongly related to RPE such that ratings are a reproducible and valid indicator of intensity of steady-state exercise. On the 15-point Borg scale of perceived exertion shown in Table 4.4, a rating of 12–13 (equivalent to 3–4 on the modified Borg scale, Table 4.5) corresponds to approximately 60% of the heart rate range or VO_{2peak}. A rating of 16 corresponds to approximately 85% of either. Most patients should therefore be exercising so that they describe the effort as between 'somewhat hard' and 'hard'. This system can usefully be introduced to patients in preparation for home-based exercise; they need to become aware of the rating they would give to exercise known from heart rate monitoring to be within the correct range. It is not suitable for a minority of individuals who persistently under-rate the intensity of their exercise.

Intensity: use of metabolic values

Finally, the intensity of exercise may be regulated by choice of activities according to their known MET (metabolic equivalents) levels. The principle that 40–85% of VO_{2peak} is adhered to is important, and prior knowledge of individual functional capacity is essential. Table 4.6 gives typical MET values for a variety of modes of exercise. External factors, such as conditions underfoot or gradients, will increase the oxygen cost of an activity above the designated value and allowance should be made for this.

Table 4.6 Typical MET values for a range of exercise modes. (Modified from ACSM (1991)[2] and Ainsworth *et al.* (1993)[6].)

Activity	Mean	Range
Cycling		
Pleasure or to work		3.0–8.0+
10 mph	7.0	
Dancing		
Social		3.7–7.4
Aerobic		6.0–9.0
Golf (carrying clubs)	5.5	
Jogging/running		
12 min/mile	8.7	
10 min/mile	10.2	
8 min/mile	12.5	
6 min/mile	16.3	
Rowing (moderate effort)	7.0	
Skipping		
60–80 skips/min	9.0	
120–140 skips/min		11.0–12.0
Squash		8.0–12.0+
Soccer		5.0–12.0+
Swimming		4.0–8.0+
Table tennis	4.1	3.0–5.0
Tennis	6.5	4.0–9.0+
Walking		
2.0 mph (30 min/mile), slow	2.5	
3.0 mph (20 min/mile), moderate	3.5	
3.5 mph (17 min/mile), brisk	4.0	
4.0 mph (15 min/mile), very brisk	4.0	
4.5 mph (13.20 min/mile), fast	4.5	
Hiking in open country		3.0–7.0

Frequency

Because some of the beneficial metabolic effects appear to be short-lived, cardiac patients should exercise frequently – even daily (for optimal benefit) – at a moderate level. There will be interactions with intensity and duration and these are likely to change over time. For individuals with very low functional capacities who cannot sustain exercise for more than a few minutes, more than one short (5 minutes) bout a day may be advisable. Typically, patients whose functional capacities exceed 5 METS should probably exercise at least 3 times a week. To avoid muscle soreness, it is advisable to have a day of rest between exercise days, at least during the first weeks of rehabilitation.

Duration

The duration of the conditioning period (exclusive of warm-up and cool-down) needs to be short initially but increased progressively to, typically, 20–30 minutes – although some individuals will wish and be able to build up further.

Rate of progression

The rate at which patients progress through a programme will vary greatly between individuals and it is an important feature of good exercise prescription that progress is monitored on an individual basis. If allowed to progress too quickly there is an increased risk of cardiovascular complications. Moreover, if the patient associates increased activity levels with discomfort rather than an acceptable sense of exertion, the likelihood of long-term compliance is reduced. Ideally, serial exercise testing will form the basis on which the prescription is modified in order to maintain the training stimulus. Where this is not the case, heart rate monitoring and rating of perceived exertion may be used to establish the appropriateness of increasing the intensity and/or duration of the selected exercise modes.

Strength training

For many patients, endurance exercise, providing a range of different muscle groups are trained, will confer 'good enough' levels of strength for the activities of daily living. For others, however, some specific training to improve strength may be indicated. The concept of individualized exercise prescription entails identifying those individuals who, for vocational or recreational reasons, will benefit from the addition of resistance training to their regimen.

When muscles are specifically trained by contracting against a high resistance, the cross-sectional area of individual fibres, and the muscle as a whole, increases – with corresponding improvements in strength. In the past, isometric exercise (which maximizes strength gains) was considered to be contraindicated because of the marked increases in left ventricular pressures and the arrhythmias which were provoked. More recently it has been demonstrated that strength can be increased safely through isometric and resistive exercise, providing that the intensity of such exercise is kept low[19]. All patients should, however, achieve a background of endurance training (ideally, a minimum of several months) before attempting to improve strength. Where this is desired, a low-resistance, high-repetition schedule should be followed to stimulate a degree of muscle hypertrophy whilst keeping the exercise-induced rise in blood pressure to a minimum. Upper body strength is likely to be important to prepare for return to manual occupational work but because of the potential for blood pressure increases, needs particular care.

Phases of exercise rehabilitation

Phase One: In-patient phase

The main purpose of exercise therapy during the in-patient phase is to counteract the deleterious effects of prolonged bed rest and in many cases the debilitating effects of long-term inactivity prior to admission. Activities include general range of motion exercises and tasks of daily living such as sitting, standing and walking. Activities performed during Phase One typically do not exceed 2–3 METs.

Phase Two: Immediate out-patient phase

During this phase activities should be designed to increase functional capacity and endurance gradually and progressively. Patients are initially encouraged to walk in and around their homes and then to walk outdoors, avoiding extremes of temperature. As functional capacity improves, rating of perceived exertion or pulse monitoring should be used to monitor the response to increases in speed or distance.

Phase Three: Intermediate out-patient phase

Clinic-based programmes typically start within 3–8 weeks of discharge from hospital and complement (rather than replace) continued efforts to increase daily physical activity levels, largely through walking. Graded exercise-testing performed prior to enrolment enables exercise prescription to be individualized. Safe and effective progression is achieved by increasing the frequency and duration of selected activities, first, and only then the intensity.

During the early stages of exercise training, extended periods of warm-up and cool-down are recommended, and the conditioning phase should represent 60–75% of predicted age-adjusted heart rate, or (if known) maximal heart rate; perhaps points 11–12 on the Borg 15-point RPE scale, or 3–4 on the modified scale. With time, and ideally following a further graded exercise test, the training heart rate may be increased to 70–85% of predicted or actual maximum.

Patients should not be discomforted nor take a long time to recover from a session; these are signs of inadequate physiological adaptation arising from too much exercise, or exercise at too high an intensity. It cannot be over-emphasized that progression must be on an individual basis and symptoms taken into consideration. It will probably need to be slower in older individuals, whose specific needs are summarized later in this chapter.

Swimming may be introduced during Phase Three but is not recommended until 6–8 weeks of rehabilitation have been completed when sternum and leg incisions in the surgery patient and heart tissue in the MI patient have had sufficient time to heal. For patients with poor technique, MET values may be much higher than indicated in standard tables.

Competitive games and exercise-to-music classes are not recommended since their intensity is dictated, at least in part, by factors not under the control of the individual participant.

Phase Four: Progression to community-based exercise programmes and long-term maintenance

Phase Four progresses or maintains the conditioning programme initiated in Phase Three and is vital if patients are to gain long-term benefit; only habitual exercise over months and years is likely to contribute to a reduction in the progression of the underlying coronary atherosclerosis and hence secondary prevention. Participants should be clinically stable, capable of regulating their own exercise prescription and have a minimal functional capacity of 5 METs, which is equivalent to walking at a speed of 4 mph without undue difficulty. Exercise prescription will be similar to that recommended for healthy adults, although activities performed in competitive circumstances should be undertaken with caution (see Table 4.7).

Structure of an exercise session

Whether working with apparently healthy individuals or in a clinical context, the format of an exercise session should include a pre-activity assessment followed by a warm-up, a conditioning (or training) phase and a cool-down. This applies equally to exercise undertaken within a supervised group setting or as part of an individual home-based prescription. For information about exercise facilities, see p. 33.

Pre-activity assessment

Participants should be assessed individually prior to exercise. This will include

Table 4.7 Guidelines for exercise prescription for cardiac patients as compared with healthy adults

Prescription	Phase I (in-patient)	Phase II (early out-patient)	Phase III (intermediate out-patient)	Phase IV (long-term maintenance)	Healthy adults
Activity	Sitting, standing, walking and ROM exercises	ADLs <4 METS Walking	Walking, cycling, swimming and supervised training	All endurance activities and light resistance training	All endurance activities, weight training and competitive sport
Frequency	2–3 × daily	Daily	3–5 × per week (walking on days when not participating in other formalized activity)	3–5 × per week	3–5 × per week
Intensity	MI & CABG RHR + 20 bpm 2–3 METs	MI & CABG RHR + 20 <4 METs RPE 11–12	60–75% HRmax (initially) increasing to 70–85% HRmax RPE 12–15	60–85% HRmax RPE 12–15	60–85% HRmax RPE 12–16
Duration	5–20 min	5–30 min	30–60 min	30–60 min	30–60 min

Note: ADL = Activity of daily living; CABG = coronary artery bypass graft surgery patient; HRmax = maximal heart rate; MET = Metabolic equivalent; MI = myocardial infarction patient; RHR = resting heart rate (bpm); ROM = range of movement; RPE = rating of perceived exertion. (Adapted from Pollock, M.L. and Wilmore, J.H. (1990) *Exercise in Health and Disease: Evaluation and Prescription for Prevention and Rehabilitation*, Philadelphia: W.B. Saunders Co.)

heart rate and blood pressure checks and questions about recent or worrying symptoms and changes in medication. In the absence of supervision, e.g. home-based exercise, the individual should be made thoroughly familiar with the use of ratings of perceived exertion, symptoms of over-exertion and circumstances in which exercise is contraindicated, including febrile illness, chest pain and ortho-paedic problems.

Warm-up

The warm-up is a period of gentle activity lasting 10–15 minutes which allows the body to adjust to a state of readiness for the ensuing exercise. Warm-up usually falls into one of two categories: Specific warm-ups to mimic the movements of the prescribed mode of activity at low intensity levels, e.g. gentle walking preceding brisker walking or jogging; and a general warm-up before a session based on a variety of exercise modalities traditionally incorporating three elements in preparation for the conditioning phase:

(1) The major joints are mobilized by taking each through a slightly greater-than-normal range of movement, e.g. the shoulders are raised and lowered, circled backwards and forwards, lumbar and thoracic sections of the spine are mobilized by sideways bending and turning behind.
(2) Metabolic demand is gradually increased by using large muscle groups in rhythmic dynamic movements, e.g. marching on the spot, stepping from side to side.
(3) The main muscle groups which will be used in the conditioning phase are stretched; each stretch position is maintained statically for about 8 seconds.

It is generally recommended that during the warm-up phase participants should achieve a heart rate within 20 bpm of the prescribed training (target) heart rate. When a participant's functional capacity is very low, even range of movement activities will represent a relatively major increase in metabolic demand, and consequently care must be taken to ensure that the warm-up fulfils its intended function of preparation and does not constitute (for some debilitated individuals) a period of training! A general warm-up suitable for a cardiac rehabilitation (CR) class is described in Appendix 3.

Warming up has been shown to enhance performance. The practice of incorporating static stretching prior to exercise has been demonstrated to reduce the incidence of musculoskeletal injuries. For cardiac patients, however, the most important consideration is that warming up appears to extend the anginal/ischaemic threshold. *Strenuous exertion without previous warm-up produces ischaemic ST-segment changes and arrhythmias, even in healthy individuals, as well as a reduction in left ventricular ejection fraction.* A warm-up period eliminates or reduces such abnormal responses.

Conditioning phase

The main objective of exercise prescription in cardiac rehabilitation is to improve functional capacity and endurance. The conditioning phase is therefore devoted predominantly to endurance activities. Selection of the most appropriate training activity and the prescribed regimen will, however, depend on the specific objectives and ability of each participant.

Continuous vs interval training

Endurance activities vary in the precision with which exercise intensity may be prescribed. Walking and stepping are examples of activities which permit precise prescription since the intensity of the activity may be controlled by adjusting walking speed or stepping height and rate. In addition, they are activities which require minimal skill, so consequently there is little individual difference in the mechanical efficiency with which they are performed. In contrast, the energy expenditure during free-moving activities such as skipping, performing jumping jacks (jumping-type movements) or rebounding on a 'mini' trampoline is highly variable and dependent on skill (hence mechanical efficiency) and motivation. In the early stages of rehabilitation, it is prudent to rely on activities which can be performed at prescribed workloads.

The type of activity used for conditioning may adopt a continuous or interval approach. Continuous training, as the name implies, involves uninterrupted activity, usually performed at a constant sub-maximal intensity. Walking, jogging, cycling, bench-stepping, rowing and swimming are all activities which lend themselves to continuous training. The advantage of this is the ease with which intensity may be prescribed and monitored. Interval training entails bouts of relatively intense work separated by periods of rest or lower level activity. The main advantage is that the total volume of work accomplished can be greater than when exercise is continuous; consequently the stimulus to physiological change is greater. It is recommended that interval training ($> 70\%$ VO_{2peak}) is only introduced once the patient has the capacity to sustain continuous low-intensity exercise (e.g. $60–70\%$ VO_{2peak}), such as walking.

Circuit training

Circuit interval training, in which the participant performs different activities at a series of stations, has become increasingly popular for cardiac rehabilitation purposes. The variety helps motivation and a number of patients can take supervised exercise in a relatively small space. The use of multiple stations gives opportunities for both upper- and lower-limb muscles to be exercised and some resistance training can be added to the dynamic activity when/if this is desirable. Consequently it is a valuable preparation for resuming both leisure and occupational activities of daily life. A circuit suitable for inclusion in a CR programme is outlined in Appendix 4. The suggested circuit is based on the simplest facilities being available, and can, of course, be adapted to take advantage of more elaborate facilities or in response to individual or group needs.

Cool-down

This is essentially active recovery and should last between 3 and 10 minutes; the greater the intensity of the preceding activity the longer is the period required to re-adjust to a non-active state. The level of activity is gradually diminished, e.g. jogging is reduced to walking and walking to marking time on the spot. This prevents blood pooling in the lower extremities when activity ceases and minimizes the possibility of post-exercise hypotension. Maintaining gentle activity also reduces the risk of cardiac arrhythmias which can, in high-risk individuals, result from high plasma catecholamine levels during the post-exercise period. Cardiac events do sometimes occur during early recovery and participants should be supervised for 10–15 minutes after completion of the exercise session.

Stretching of the major muscle groups involved in the conditioning phase helps alleviate delayed onset muscle soreness. The stretches performed as part of the warm-up should be repeated in the recovery phase. For detailed information about the role and execution of stretches in recovery and in the attainment of improved flexibility, the reader is referred to a number of specialized texts[20,21].

Exercise for special groups of patients

Until fairly recently, exercise training and even regular moderate physical activity were discouraged in patients with certain cardiac conditions. It was thought that angina, as opposed to a patient with stable and healed myocardial infarction, could be made unstable by exercise. Similarly, there was a fear that exercise may worsen heart failure and left ventricular dysfunction. Both of these conditions are now recognized as responding favourably to exercise training in stable patients. Certain training effects are beneficial, including a reduction in heart rate and blood pressure at sub-maximal workloads, and an improvement in peripheral vascular and possibly coronary vascular function.

Older patients

The benefits conferred by exercise training in young cardiac patients may also be expected in the elderly, and older cardiac patients should therefore be encouraged to participate in exercise programmes. The general principles governing the development of exercise prescription (outlined earlier in the chapter) are applicable to older patients, but where individual prescription is concerned, it must be recognized that in this group functional capacity is reduced, partly due to age-related changes, and partly due to decreased habitual physical activity levels. In addition, exercise prescription may be complicated by the increased incidence of osteoporosis, hypertension, orthostatic hypotension, and diabetes mellitus. Vulnerability to musculoskeletal injury as a result of muscle atrophy will also be increased. Some modification to standard exercise programming is therefore appropriate.

Endurance training should be initiated at a low percentage of peak work capacity. Training intensities as low as 30–40% peak oxygen consumption have been shown to improve functional capacity in older individuals, and exercising at comfortable levels is associated with greater safety and improved compliance. To minimize the potential for musculoskeletal complications, endurance training should *exclude* high-impact activities, and resistance training should be accomplished by using lighter weights but higher repetitions than those typically prescribed for younger patients.

The cool-down period should be extended to allow for the longer time that exercising heart rates take to return to pre-exercise rates, and the greater risk of venous pooling owing to age-related slowing of the baroreceptor responsiveness. Exercise in hot or humid environments should be avoided, since the ability to dissipate heat is often impaired in the elderly. Finally, there is a need for increased supervision to prevent falls arising from orthostatic hypotension. For a fuller discussion of the specific needs of elderly cardiac patients, the reader is referred to Williams[22].

Angina

Before recommending exercise as a therapy for angina patients, it is necessary first to stabilize the condition and optimize therapy; only when the patient's angina is stable and uncomplicated should exercise be advised. Contraindications to exercise therapy include: unstable symptoms, recent-onset or rest pains, and a very positive low-level (first stage of Bruce protocol) exercise test suggesting the possibility of left main-stem or proximal triple vessel coronary artery disease better managed by a revascularization procedure.

In suitable patients, training has been shown to increase exercise tolerance, prolong the time to ischaemic ECG changes, reduce the frequency and severity of angina, and possibly promote the growth of collateral vessel formation within the myocardium. In addition, other training effects on cardiac risk factors would be beneficial in this patient group including reductions in cholesterol, increases in HDL cholesterol, reductions in fibrinogen levels, and reductions in sympathetic tone and arterial blood pressure. Overviews of CR programmes including a component of exercise training have suggested a net reduction in long-term mortality in patients with CHD recovering from an MI[23,24].

Heart failure

Patients with heart failure may be limited by dyspnoea or fatigue at very low work-loads, and at first it might be thought they would be unable to exercise enough to obtain any training effects. However, recent studies have shown that even quite severely affected patients with class II-III symptoms [New York Heart Association classes indicating symptoms on exercise well below usual physical exertion] can benefit. Benefits include increased exercise tolerance, reduced sympathetic drive, improved ventilatory efficiency and less dyspnoea, and an improvement in peripheral blood flow and skeletal muscle function. All of these factors are thought to explain the improvement in patients' quality of life reported after training, and some may have a good effect on disease progression[25].

Training patients with heart failure is a specialist area at present as these patients require particular stabilization and assessment prior to commencing training (see also Chapter 3). It is essential to optimize therapy to recommend training only when the patient's condition is stable and when there are no signs of acute decompensation, such as pulmonary or peripheral oedema. In addition, silent ventricular arrhythmias in this condition are common and it is important to exclude serious exercise-induced ventricular arrhythmias. The choice of exercise type and level needs to be highly individualized to take into account the exercise tolerance of each patient, and patients may need to have their programmes re-evaluated on a regular basis depending on their clinical course. Despite these limitations, these patients are a particularly satisfying group for whom to prescribe exercise therapy, as even small increases in exercise efficiency and tolerance can have dramatic effects on the ability to perform everyday activities and hence improve quality of life and the possibility of independent self-care.

Arrhythmias

This is one of the most difficult areas in exercise therapy. Although there is good evidence that training can help prevent serious ventricular arrhythmias in animal models and in some human studies, there remains the concern that, prior to realizing the beneficial effects of training, there may be acute hazards from individual bouts of exercise. In patients with unstable, prolonged or complex ventricular arrhythmias most cardiologists would advise against any significant exercise. Once the arrhythmia has been controlled, by drug therapy, revascular-ization or by electrophysiological ablation, this restriction could be removed. Despite this concern, however, we might be producing more hazard than benefit if we prevent increased fitness in a larger group with stable and non-life-threatening arrhythmias. Increased fitness is associated with lower resting sympathetic nervous tone and enhanced vagal tone, both of which may protect against serious arrhythmias.

Although this area remains clouded in uncertainty, it would seem prudent to monitor all maximal exercise tests carefully and only encourage regular exercise in those patients who do not demonstrate exercise-induced ventricular arrhythmias. Regular monitoring of all exercise sessions is sometimes recommended, partly for medicolegal reasons, but eventually patients need to know if they can continue moderate exercise at home in unmonitored circumstances. The rate of serious arrhythmias in well-evaluated patients who have undergone multiple monitored exercise tests without complication is extremely low, and probably less than the rate of unexpected arrhythmias and events occurring in this patient population at any time of the day. This remains an area where further research is urgently needed.

Summary of key points

- The objectives of exercise testing are various: diagnostic; prognostic; to evaluate therapy, functional capacity and specific exercise-induced responses.
- The protocol to be adopted, and end-points selected, will be determined by the test objectives.
- The diagnostic power of exercise testing is increased by the addition of perfusion or functional imaging, which provides independent evidence of the significance of ECG changes.
- Certain medical conditions increase the risk of exercise testing and should be considered relative or absolute contraindications to maximal exercise testing.
- Exercise training in CHD patients results in increased peak oxygen uptake and thereby reduces the physiological stress of tasks of everyday life.
- Exercise training has a salutary effect on the major modifiable CHD risk factors.
- Endurance training should be the major component of the exercise regimen for CHD patients.
- Individualized exercise prescription takes account of the mode, intensity, duration and frequency of exercise, and incorporates the special needs of different groups, such as older people.
- Exercise training must incorporate warm-up, conditioning, and cool-down phases.

References

1. Gibbons, I., Blair, S.N., Kohl, H.W. and Cooper, K. (1980) The safety of maximal exercise testing, *Circulation*, **80**, 846–52.
2. American College of Sports Medicine (1991) *Guidelines for Exercise Testing and Prescription*, Philadelphia: Lea and Febiger.
3. Froelicher, V.F., Duarte, G.M., Oakes, D.F., *et al.* (1989) The prognostic value of the exercise test, *Disease a Month* **34**, 677–735.
4. Krone, R.J., Dwyer, E.J., Greenberg, H., *et al.* (1989) Risk stratification in patients with first non-Q-wave infarctions: limited value of the early low-level

exercise test after uncomplicated infarcts, The Multicenter Post-Infarction Research Group, *Journal of the American College of Cardiology*, **14**, 31–7.

5. CASS principle investigators and their associates. (1984) Myocardial infarction and mortality in the Coronary Artery Surgery Study (CASS) randomized trial, *New England Journal of Medicine*, **310**, 750.

6. Ainsworth, B.E., Haskell, W.L., Leon, A.S., Jacobs, D.R., Montoye, H.J., Sallis, J.F. and Paffenbarger, R.S. (1993) Compendium of physical activities: classification of energy costs of human physical activities, *Medicine and Science in Sports and Exercise*, **25**, 71–80.

7. Singh, S., Morgan, M.D.L. and Hardman, A.E. (1992) The development of the shuttle walking test of disability in patients with chronic airways obstruction, *Thorax*, **47**, 1019–24.

8. Borg, G.A. (1973) Perceived exertion: a note on history and methods, *Medicine and Science in Sports and Exercise*, **5**, 90–3.

9. Borg, G. (1982) A category scale with ratio properties for intermodal and interindividual comparisons. In H.G. Geissler and P. Petzoid (eds) *Psychophysical Judgment and the Process of Perception*, Berlin: VEB Deutscher Verlag der Wissenschaften.

10. Leon, A.S., Certo, C., Comoss, P., Franklin, B.A., Froelicher, V., Haskell, W.L., Hellerstein, H.K., Marley, W.P., Pollock, M.L., Ries, A., Froelicher Sivarajan, E. and Smith, L.K. (1990) Position statement of the American Association of Cardiovascular and Pulmonary Rehabilitation. Scientific evidence of the value of cardiac rehabilitation services with emphasis on patients following myocardial infarction Section 1: Exercise conditioning component, *Journal of Cardiopulmonary Rehabilitation*, **10**, 79–87.

11. Saltin, B. and Rowell, L.B. (1980) Functional adaptations to physical activity and inactivity, *Federation Proceedings*, **39**, 1506–13.

12. Arroll, B. and Beaglehole, R. (1992) Does physical activity lower blood pressure: a critical review of the clinical trials, *Journal of Clinical Epidemiology*, **45(5)**, 439–47.

13. Ehsani, A.A., Biello, D.R., Schultz, J., Sobel, B.E. and Holloszy, J.O. (1986) Improvement of left ventricular contractile function in patients with coronary artery disease, *Circulation*, **74**, 350–88.

14. Van Camp, S.P. and Peterson, R.A. (1986) Cardiovascular complications of outpatient cardiac rehabilitation programmes, *Journal of the American Medical Association*, **256**, 1160–3.

15. Haskell, W.L. (1994) Health consequences of physical activity: understanding and challenges regarding dose-response, *Medicine and Science in Sports and Exercise*, **26**, 649–60.

16. Willich, S.N., Lewis, M., Löwel, H., Arntz, J-R., Schubert, F. and Schröder, R. (1993) Physical exertion as a trigger of acute myocardial infarction, *New England Journal of Medicine*, **329**, 1684–90.

17. Morris, J.N., Clayton, D.G., Everitt, M.G., Semmence, A.M. and Burgess, E.H. (1990) Exercise in leisure time: coronary attack and death rates, *British*

Heart Journal, **63**, 325–34.

18. Wenger, N.K. (1991) Rehabilitation of the coronary patient: a preview of tomorrow, *Journal of Cardiopulmonary Rehabilitation*, **11**, 93–8.

19. Vander, L.B., Franklin, B.A., Wrisley, D. and Ruberfire, M. (1986) Acute cardiovascular responses to Nautilus exercise in cardiac patients; implications for exercise training, *Annals of Sports Medicine*, **2**, 165–9.

20. Smith, B. (1994) *Flexibility for Sport*, Marlborough, Wilts.: Crowood Press.

21. Corbin, C.B., *et al.* (1987) *Staying Flexible*, Amsterdam: Time-Life Books.

22. Williams, M.A. (1994) *Exercise Testing and Training in the Elderly Cardiac Patient*, Champaign, Illinois: Human Kinetics Books.

23. O'Connor, G.T., Buring, J.E., Yusuf, S., Goldhaber, S.Z., Olmstead, E.M., Paffenbarger, R.S. and Hennekens, C.H. (1989) An overview of randomized trials of rehabilitation with exercise after myocardial infarction, *Circulation*, **80**, 234–44.

24. Oldridge, N.B., Guyatt, G.H., Fischer, M.S. and Rimm, A.A. (1988) Cardiac rehabilitation after myocardial infarction: combined experience of randomized clinical trials, *Journal of the American Medical Association*, **260**, 945–50.

25. Coats, A.J.S. (1993) Exercise rehabilitation in chronic heart failure, *Journal of the American College of Cardiology*, **22 (Suppl. A)**, 172A–177A.

Chapter 5

Enhancing Exercise Motivation and Adherence in Cardiac Rehabilitation

Summary

The health benefits associated with cardiac rehabilitation (CR) – physical and psychological – are widely acknowledged and accepted. However, adherence to CR programmes is repeatedly reported to be disappointing. Approximately 50% of those who start on exercise rehabilitation programmes can be expected to drop out within 6 to 12 months. It is important therefore to address the problem of poor adherence and investigate strategies which may help to improve compliance. Specialists and researchers in the field of exercise motivation have proposed various techniques, both practical and theoretical, in an attempt to improve compliance in CR. This chapter will examine several of these techniques.

Objectives of cardiac rehabilitation

The World Health Organization's definition of cardiac rehabilitation (CR; see p. xi) has received considerable support from researchers in the field of CR compliance, and is worthy of consideration with regard to the aims and objectives of CR programmes. The definition suggests that participants take individual responsibility for the rehabilitation process, the ultimate goal being to lead as normal a life as possible – to resume or maintain one's established pattern of living.

The question of an active and productive life will require the adoption and maintenance of life-long regular exercise behaviour. Bearing this in mind, some CR programmes may wish to consider or reassess long-term objectives. It appears that few have formalized long-term objectives. Short-term programme objectives are more commonplace and essentially relate to physiological targets, i.e. improved exercise tolerance. This may be potentially limiting if, at the same time, programme staff fail to recognize or accept long-term behaviour change goals. For example, some participants may fall well short of physiological targets, but may also have increased activity in their daily routine. This very positive outcome may receive little reinforcement. Introducing activity into the daily routine, albeit at a very low level, which becomes a life-long habit, is likely to have more long-term health benefits than adhering successfully to a supervised programme which is discontinued once physiological targets have been reached.

Cardiac rehabilitation should not be seen as a prescription course of treatment, which may be discontinued once fitness is improved. Any health improvements will be lost quickly if exercise is discontinued. Participants in CR and their partners should be made aware of this from the outset. The rehabilitative exercise programme is simply a 'helping hand' to encourage life-long behavioural change. Oldridge[1] notes that:

> ... the real benefit of exercise rehabilitation may in fact be less related to changes in exercise tolerance than to improvements in psychological well being and quality of life.

The idea of individual responsibility, as suggested in the World Health Organization definition, is consistent with a self-regulation compliance model suggested by Oldridge[2]. The model advocates the use of self-management strategies to improve compliance, and stresses the importance of individuals taking responsibility for their own rehabilitation. The participant should quickly become the primary active agent in the rehabilitative process. If the participant perceives the health professional to be in charge the long-term effectiveness of the behaviour change may be minimized. If participants perceive themselves to have equal responsibility along with the programme staff, then long-term effectiveness can probably be optimized.

Programme directors may wish to consider incorporating techniques to encourage and reinforce greater patient responsibility in a compliance-enhancing strategy. For example, involving participants in decision-making and programme setting. If CR programme staff accept the concepts contained in the World Health Organization definition, i.e. self-responsibility, return to normality and continued active role in the wider community, then it should be reflected in the objectives, philosophy and operation of the programme. It is also important to ensure that participants appreciate their significant individual responsibility in the rehabilitation process – in *their* rehabilitation process – and also understand the long-term behaviour change goals from the outset.

Compliance, adherence and drop-out

For the purposes of this chapter, 'compliance' and 'adherence' are used interchangeably and relate to the extent to which an individual's behaviour reflects health advice in relation to CR. With regard to the aims of CR, short-term goals would relate to adherence with programme objectives, whereas continued adherence to a habitual active lifestyle would be a long-term goal.

'Drop-outs' may be defined as those participants missing more than a given number or percentage of consecutive sessions (or time)[3,4,5,6]. Investigation of drop-out rates of several studies suggests that at best exercise rehabilitation programmes should expect only a 75–80% compliance rate[1,7]. Much apparent drop-out is probably unavoidable. The most prominent reason reported for unavoidable drop-out is ill health or medical complications. Oldridge[8] reported that approximately 45% who drop-out from CR fall into this category. In addition, Dishman[7] also accepts work conflicts, relocation and accessibility of the programme site as unavoidable barriers. However, it could be argued that some of those non-medical barriers may be interpreted as excuses rather than genuine barriers[9,10].

Any compliance-enhancing strategy should concentrate on addressing reasons for drop-out which may be avoidable. The most common potentially avoidable reasons given for drop-out are inaccessible exercise programme locations, inconvenient time of exercise programme, lack of time or work conflicts, and poor partner support[7]. Obviously the impact of any of these factors will vary considerably from one participant to the next, but a compliance-enhancing strategy could attempt to address at least some of these barriers at a programme level. For example, the problem of poor partner support, although highly individual, could perhaps be improved by generally fostering greater partner involvement in the rehabilitation programme. This may involve encouraging partners to attend exercise classes, educational sessions, social events, etc. If partners are aware of the tremendous potential for health gain from a structured exercise regimen and also witness their loved ones enjoying exercise in a safe, monitored environment, they are likely to become less fearful and more supportive of the programme. Depending on resources, partner education sessions can range from a one-off group information and demonstration session, to a range of meetings with relevant professionals, e.g. the dietician or psychologist from the CR programme.

An inaccessible location or inconvenient times are difficult to address, especially when resources are limited. Programme planners could investigate the possibility of providing rehabilitation sessions at different times, particularly in the evening or at weekends to facilitate access for participants who work; or provide rehabilitation sessions at more than one location, therefore making the programme accessible to a wider geographical audience. Programme staff may wish to devise their own protocol for evaluation of programme adherence. Avoidable and unavoidable drop-out as well as programme and long-term adherence criteria could be established.

For example:

Unavoidable drop-out:
- Medical complications
- Relocation

- Work conflicts
- Inaccessible programme location.

Avoidable drop-out:

- Any other reasons not included in the unavoidable dropout may be potentially avoidable.

Programme adherence:

- Attended at least 75% of the appropriate CR sessions over a 3-month period.

Long-term adherence:

- Exercising regularly and independently 18 months after beginning a CR programme.

All of these objective measures should of course be negotiated and agreed with each participant when beginning CR. This will reinforce the self-regulatory aspect and long-term nature of CR. Some programmes may wish to include the agreed measures in a written contract which is discussed later in this chapter.

Whilst considering non-compliance, it is important to consider whether a 'drop-out' is in fact a drop-out ! Although a considerable number of participants may apparently drop out of structured CR programmes, several studies suggest that a significant proportion continue to exercise on their own. In one study, 50% of 'drop-outs' from a rehabilitative programme reported to be exercising regularly on their own 12 months later[11]. With regard to long-term adherence objectives of a CR programme, this should be viewed as a positive outcome. Programme staff should accept that some people will be more suited to exercising independently than in a group environment and that programme drop-out does not automatically mean exercise drop-out.

Theoretical models and practical implications

In an attempt to improve exercise compliance within CR settings, researchers have applied well-established models and theories from general psychology. Models which have been frequently used to explain exercise behaviour are the theory of planned behaviour, the health belief model and the concept of self-efficacy.

The Theory of Planned Behaviour

The Theory of Planned Behaviour (TPB)[12] is an extension of the Theory of Reasoned Action[13] and is based upon the belief that the most important influence upon behaviour is behavioural intention – what an individual intends to do. Influencing behaviour is achieved by influencing a person's intentions. So, in order for an individual to adhere successfully to a CR programme, he or she must first *intend* whole-heartedly to do so.

Behavioural intention is affected by three factors:

- An individual's attitude towards performing the behaviour;
- Perceived subjective social norms, i.e. the degree to which significant other people feel performing this behaviour is important;
- Perceived behavioural control, i.e. the degree to which the individual feels performing a particular behaviour is under his/her control.

With regard to exercise behaviour, the attitude component could relate to an individual's belief that the exercise therapy will be effective at improving health or fitness and, in turn, the relative value of that outcome, i.e. how important health or improved fitness are to that particular individual. A review of studies which have applied components of this model in an exercise compliance context[7], describes an association between attitudes, intentions and exercise behaviour. This lends support to compliance-enhancing strategies that attempt to influence positively attitudes to the potential benefits of CR. The provision of appropriate information for participants with regard to the significant health benefits associated with exercise therapy would form part of such a strategy.

The subjective normative element of the model concerns the influence that the opinions of significant other people have on the individual, i.e. the degree to which people, e.g. doctor, nurse, partner and friends, think participation in an exercise programme is important. This element also includes the value the individual places on that particular person's approval or disapproval.

The normative belief component is consistent with considerable evidence that partner support can improve exercise programme compliance[10,11,14]. Cardiac rehabilitation staff may therefore wish to foster partner support as much as possible. For example, an educational programme for both partners and participants, which runs alongside the exercise therapy programme could link with both attitudinal and normative motivational components of this model. Enlisting the support of significant others may also prove to be fruitful. Influential health professionals, e.g. cardiologists, general practitioners, practice nurses, should be kept informed or involved in the operation and underlying philosophy of the programme. They may then be more likely to influence positively their patients' commitment with regard to the programme.

The control element relates to the amount of control individuals feel they have over their CR programme. The more control participants feel they have, the more likely are they to adhere successfully to their programme. Factors affecting perceptions of control may be internal or external. Internal factors could include: confidence in one's physical ability and skills to perform the exercise therapy, or emotional confidence in one's ability to undertake and maintain the programme. External factors could include: not having to depend on others for transport or social support, being able to avoid work or family commitments which interfere with one's ability to perform exercise rehabilitation. The participant responsibility mentioned earlier in this chapter relates to the control elements of the TPB. Because it is the cognitive elements of this model that shape behavioural intention and subsequent behavioural patterns, the TPB is most useful when applied to health behaviours that we must explicitly think about doing, e.g. taking up exercise. Behaviours which are habitual and require little thought, like smoking, for a regular smoker, are less easily changed in accordance with the proposals of the TPB.

The Health Belief Model

The Health Belief Model (HBM)[15] proposes that adherence to a particular health behaviour is influenced by an individual's perception of:

■ Vulnerability or susceptibility to the health problem;
■ The seriousness of the health problem;
■ Available and effective action to tackle the health problem;
■ Potential costs and benefits involved in undertaking the particular action.

Potential costs or 'barriers' with regard to CR could be inconvenience of the time and physical effort required to exercise. Benefits could include improved health and physical capabilities, social support, or simply enjoyment. Cardiac rehabilitation participants will continually undertake a process of cost-benefit analysis with regard to their rehabilitation programme. If the perceived costs of participating outweigh the perceived benefits, then it is unlikely that he or she will continue to adhere to the programme recommendations.

The model also recognizes the role of triggers or cues to action in shaping behaviour patterns. Cues may be internal (perception of a symptom, e.g. angina), or external (reminder or persuasion by a peer or partner). Participants in CR may be encouraged to develop cues themselves to help them maintain their adapted lifestyle, e.g. try asking relatives to support or provide reminders. Participants could also try evaluating their progress (or lack of) at the start of every month.

Self-efficacy

Self-efficacy (see also Chapter 6) is the personal belief or expectancy that one is capable of making changes successfully or of carrying out a desired behaviour[16]. If CR participants believe that they are personally capable of achieving their exercise prescription goal, then they are much more likely – so the theory suggests – to adhere to their exercise regimen than participants who may be unsure of their ability to succeed. Several factors may enhance an individual's belief that he or she can succeed. Positive reinforcement (e.g. verbal praise from programme staff), emotional persuasion (e.g. witnessing peers succeeding), physical and psychological feedback (e.g. being able to cope physically with the exercise prescription) – all help to promote self-efficacy.

Several authors advocate the practice of participants signing an agreement with regard to commitment to their exercise programme. This procedure will help to reinforce self-efficacy, particularly if participants have been involved in writing their programme and setting their own programme goals[17,18]. Oldridge and Jones[5] reported a 65% compliance rate among those who were prepared to sign an agreement. Compliance was reduced to 20% among those who were not prepared to sign the written agreement. Several studies have found greater compliance amongst patients who agree to sign a contract than those who would not.

Self-efficacy is highly specific to a particular context and is liable to change from day to day. For example, confidence in personal ability to succeed with an exercise programme could be shattered by a perceived poor performance during a rehabilitation class or by the recurrence of physical symptoms. Programme leaders should be aware of this possibility and ensure that programme goals are realistic and achievable. They should provide positive reinforcement, particularly if they witness participants having a 'bad day'. Also, feelings of efficacy may be positive in a group rehabilitation class with the immediate support of programme staff, but low with regard to exercising on their own at home. Some participants may require considerable support and encouragement to comply with their home exercise programme, and have greater confidence to carry out their home-based programme if they are able to pair up with a peer who lives nearby.

Self-efficacy should develop as participants progress with their CR programme since they come to realize their physical capabilities and experience physical improvement. This in turn is likely to affect compliance positively. However, self-efficacy needs to be actively promoted by CR staff from the outset of the programme. Staff can inadvertently promote the converse of self-efficacy, i.e. dependency, if they do not actively encourage participants to achieve goals with their own sense of involvement and achievement. In the initial stages of rehabilitation, exercise prescription should be modest enough to be achievable to enhance self-belief and self-confidence, yet sufficiently challenging to enhance physical capabilities.

All of these theories have at one time or another been used to explain and improve exercise compliance in CR. No one model or combination of models has been able to predict exercise compliance completely. When one considers that theoretical models are attempting to explain something as individual and complex as human behaviour, this apparent failure is perhaps not surprising. The models do, however, include some valuable predictive elements with practical application, which could usefully be included in a compliance-enhancing strategy.

Other compliance-enhancing techniques

Relapse prevention

It is likely that many participants will at one time or another fail to comply with aspects of their CR programme. It is possible to reduce the effect of relapse by planning for such occasions in advance. Participants should be encouraged to plan for likely triggers for relapse, e.g. holidays, moving house, unexpected events, etc. This exercise will help to put any relapse into perspective, i.e. a temporary pause in the rehabilitative programme. Participants should be made aware that programme staff will not view temporary relapse as failure and will be happy to revise individual programmes if necessary and welcome them back to the group.

'Buddy' support

Some experts suggest pairing up newcomers with experienced veterans and encouraging the veteran or 'graduate' to take the newcomer 'under his or her wing'[10]. Newcomers may find they are able to relate easily to 'graduates' who have themselves experienced cardiac problems. 'Graduates' are also likely to have an empathic understanding of the possible fears and insecurities beginners may experience when embarking on a CR programme. 'Graduates' can provide a sensitive introduction to the new social environment, inform newcomers what they might expect, provide positive reinforcement and perhaps telephone newcomers should they miss sessions.

Summary of key points

Compliance-enhancing techniques

The most appropriate compliance-enhancing techniques will depend upon: the philosophy, objectives and operational logistics of the programme; available resources; programme staff; and most importantly the circumstances, personality and the social, emotional and physiological needs of each participant.

Compliance-enhancing techniques are divided into three sections:

(1) Strategies to consider with regard to initiation, adoption and development of an exercise rehabilitation programme;
(2) Strategies to consider with regard to exercise programme maintenance; and
(3) General programme strategies.

Initiation, adoption and development strategies

■ Where appropriate, encourage participants to take individual responsibility for their rehabilitation processes;
■ Set realistic, achievable exercise programmes involving each participant in the process of programme setting. Negotiate and agree the programme goals;

- If appropriate, encourage each participant to sign an agreement or contract;
- Encourage 'graduates' or experienced programme participants to adopt and support newcomers;
- Ensure that each participant has reasonable and realistic expectations;
- Inform participants in advance of possible side-effects of exercise therapy, such as tiredness and post-exercise muscle soreness.

Programme maintenance strategies

- Revise and progress individual programmes regularly;
- Constantly reinforce the importance of daily home-based exercises;
- Encourage participants to keep records of daily activities which are reported regularly;
- Constantly reinforce the benefits, both physical and psychological, of exercise rehabilitation;
- Continually encourage partner involvement and support. Include partners in exercise programmes, educational sessions and social events;
- Prepare participants in advance for 'bad' days or relapses;
- Provide regular positive feedback and reinforcement.

General programme strategies

- Consider providing exercise opportunities at more than one venue and at different times during the day;
- Involve participants or participant representatives in all major programme decisions.

References

1. Oldridge, N.B. (1988) Cardiac rehabilitation exercise programme: compliance and compliance-enhancing strategies, *Sports Medicine*, **6**, 42–55.
2. Oldridge, N.B. (1988) Compliance in exercise in cardiac rehabilitation. In R.K. Dishman (ed.), *Exercise Adherence*, Champaign, Illinois: Human Kinetics Books, pp. 283–304.
3. Blumenthal, J.A., Williams, S., Wallace, A.G., Williams, R.B. and Needles, T.L. (1982) Physiological and psychological variables predict compliance to prescribed exercise therapy in patients recovering from myocardial infarction, *Psychosomatic Medicine*, **44**, 519–27.
4. Daltroy, L.H. (1985) Improving cardiac patient adherence to exercise regimes: A clinical trial of health education, *Journal of Cardiopulmonary Rehabilitation*, **5**, 40–9.
5. Oldridge, N.B. and Jones, N.L. (1983) Improving patient compliance in

cardiac exercise rehabilitation: Effects of written agreement and self-monitoring, *Journal of Cardiac Rehabilitation*, **3**, 257–62.

6. Oldridge, N.B., Donner, A., Buck, C., Andrew, G. and Jones, N.L. (1983) Prognostic indices of dropout from the Ontario exercise-heart collaborative study, *American Journal of Cardiology*, **51**, 70–4.

7. Dishman, R.K. (1986) Exercise compliance: a new view for public health, *The Physician and Sports Medicine*, **14**, 5.

8. Oldridge, N.B. (1991) Compliance with cardiac rehabilitation services, *Journal of Cardiopulmonary Rehabilitation*, **11**, 115–27.

9. Rejeski, W.J. (1992) Motivation for exercise behaviour: a critique of theoretical direction. In G.C. Roberts (ed.), *Understanding Motivation In Sport and Exercise*, Champaign, Illinois: Human Kinetics Books, pp. 129–57.

10. Rejeski, W.J. and Hobson, M. (1994) A framework for enhancing exercise motivation in rehabilitative medicine. In Quinney Gauvin Wall (eds), *Toward Active Living*, Champaign, Illinois: Human Kinetics Books, pp. 107–113.

11. Oldridge, N.B. and Spencer, J. (1985) Exercise habits and perceptions before and after graduating or drop-out from supervised cardiac exercise rehabilitation, *Journal of Cardiopulmonary Rehabilitation*, **5**, 313–9.

12. Ajzen, I. (1991) The theory of planned behaviour, *Behaviour and Human Decision Process*, **50**, 179–211.

13. Fishbein, M. and Ajzen, I. (1975) *Beliefs, Attitude, Intention and Behaviour: An Introduction to Theory and Research Reading*, Philadelphia: Addison-Wesley.

14. Erling, J. and Oldridge, N.B. (1985) Effect of a spousal support programme on compliance with cardiac rehabilitation, *Medicine and Science in Sports and Exercise*, **17(2)**, 284.

15. Becker, M.H. (ed.) (1974) The health belief model and personal health behaviour, *Health Education Monograph*, **2**.

16. Bandura, A. (1977) Self efficacy: toward a unifying theory of behavioural change, *Psychological Review*, **84**, 191–215.

17. Oldridge, N.B. and Streiner, D.L. (1990) The health belief model: predicting compliance and drop-out in cardiac rehabilitation, *Medicine and Science in Sports and Exercise*, **22**, 678–83.

18. American College of Sports Medicine (1991) Methods for changing health behaviours. In: *Guidelines For Exercise Testing and Prescription*, Philadelphia: Lea and Febiger, Chapter 4, pp. 187–99.

Chapter 6

Psychosocial Aspects of Cardiac Rehabilitation

Summary

This chapter outlines the psychological experiences and difficulties of cardiac patients and describes the role of psychosocial intervention in the cardiac rehabilitation setting. Cardiac rehabilitation programmes must provide an explicit focus on psychosocial issues if optimal quality of life and lifestyle management are to be achieved by patients.

Introduction

Diagnosis of coronary disease has major psychological consequences whether the diagnosis comes in the aftermath of an acute coronary event, such as a myocardial infarction (MI), or in relation to angina or other cardiac problems necessitating medication, further testing or surgery[1]. Much of the clinical and research work on cardiac rehabilitation (CR) has been with middle-aged men from Western cultures who have experienced myocardial infarction. However, there is evidence that groups with other clinical problems can be assisted by CR. For instance, in patients with angina pectoris, a primary goal is the management of pain and the associated limitations in activities of daily living. Stress management training has been shown to significantly lower patients' experience of pain[2,3]. This may be an important consideration for patients who are either unwilling to, or precluded from, participating in the exercise component of CR. One UK study of note demonstrates how psychosocial improvement can be achieved for patients with the use of a standardized training manual – *The Heart Manual*. Developed and tested in Scotland[4], this manual to assist cardiac patients in a phased return to daily activities has been shown to improve psychosocial functioning and reduce health service use in the year following myocardial infarction.

Many different psychological reactions are experienced by cardiac patients. A typical psychological response in the first days following an MI is for the patient to deny that the MI has actually occurred. This early denial is usually followed by an awareness of the events and a period of anxiety and depression. Denial, if not prolonged, may provide an early protection for the patient who would otherwise be overwhelmed and be unable to come to terms with the meaning of recent events. Equally, a period of anxiety and depression following MI or news of a serious cardiac condition should be viewed as a normal reaction to such a major stressful life event (in the same way that depression, for instance, is a feature of bereavement following the death of a significant other). Approximately one-third to one-half of patients experience anxiety and depression following an MI[5,6]. In the long term, however, unchecked anxiety and depression can prevent patients from achieving a full return to daily activities. Patients with psychological problems have been found to be less likely to return to former employment, less likely to adopt or maintain recommended lifestyle changes and less likely to return to adequate sexual relations. Depression, in particular, has also been linked with increased risk of mortality following MI[7].

A major cardiac event has psychological implications beyond the patient. Family members, particularly partners, are profoundly affected by a patient's coronary condition[8]. They may experience a range of symptoms from guilt (concerning onset of the patient's condition) to anger (that the patient or the condition is disrupting family lifestyle or personal plans). They may feel both responsibility for the future welfare of the patient and fear of that responsibility.

Awareness of the range of psychological reactions following an acute coronary event allows us to target key difficulties by psychological intervention in the cardiac setting. A number of key points need to be emphasized in advance. These are:

- A significant proportion of psychological distress following a coronary episode does *not* resolve spontaneously over time[9].
- Exercise training alone is generally *not* effective as a means of restoring psychological functioning[10].
- The primary goal of cardiac rehabilitation – for most patients, especially in future clinical populations – will not be to extend life but rather to reduce morbidity and increase quality of life. Resolution of psychological difficulties is a major contributor to improved quality of life for cardiac patients[11].
- Resolution of psychological difficulties increases the likelihood that other goals in cardiac rehabilitation, e.g. increased exercise, decreased smoking and alcohol, and dietary and medication adherence, are managed successfully[12].

Psychological interventions

Since cardiac events are associated with a range of negative psychological reactions, it is important first to clarify a patient's understanding of cardiac illness and the individual meaning of the event for that person. Clarification of the nature of heart disease is important for subsequent efforts by the rehabilitation team to change lifestyle factors such as diet and smoking. Following this, specific management of affective response generated by the cardiac event can be addressed. The management of lifestyle changes, such as stress reduction, is a key component of psychological intervention. The goals of, and specific details on, psychological interventions are described next.

Goals of psychological intervention in cardiac rehabilitation

The goals of psychological intervention are to:

(1) *Increase quality of life* – by:
  ■ Reducing negative psychological reactions, such as anxiety and depression (**Emotions management**)
  ■ Increasing the likelihood of return to former activities, such as employment, social life and sexual relationships (**Role restoration**) and
(2) *Promote secondary prevention* – by:
  ■ Increasing knowledge and clarifying misperceptions about heart disease and its management (**Knowledge**)
  ■ Increasing motivation for, and adoption and maintenance of, a healthy lifestyle (**Motivation; Skills development and maintenance**).

The management of each of these is considered as they would be addressed in temporal sequence in the CR setting.

Knowledge

Goals:
■ Establishment of a shared understanding of cardiac disease by professionals and patients – resulting in
■ Increased motivation to undertake CR activities.

Education about heart disease should start in the coronary care unit (CCU) and continue through the patient's hospital stay. However, given the range of emotional reactions expected at this time and the ever-reducing length of in-patient stay in hospital, it is reasonable to expect that many patients will not remember significant proportions of information. In this regard, written information can be particularly useful as it is available to patient and family when *they* are ready to focus on the matter and concentrate on particular details. An outline of the out-patient CR programme – if explained briefly to patients during hospitalization and supplemented with a short information leaflet – is likely to encourage patients to participate in the programme.

[Many excellent examples of such written information exist. For those preparing written information, Ley[13] provides clear guidelines on effective methods of communicating written information.]

Even with the provision of information during the patient's stay in hospital, it is important to start the psychological component of CR with a section on knowledge. Inappropriate beliefs or assumptions can hinder the whole rehabilitation process. For instance, if patients believe that 'stress' alone caused their MI or other cardiac problem (and many do), they may be unwilling to adopt dietary or other lifestyle changes.

Therefore discussion on heart disease should focus on the following points:

- What causes heart disease?
  (Risk factors for MI, etc.)
- What happens in heart disease?
  (MI, CABG, PTCA; the meaning and cause of pain, etc.)
- What are the consequences of having heart disease?
  (Rest and recovery period, risk of subsequent events, secondary prevention, effects on work, social and sexual activities).

A useful framework for eliciting patient views on heart disease or specific events such as MI is the following:

- Label/symptoms
  (Name and associated symptoms: e.g. do patients believe one can have an MI without severe pain?)
- Time-line
  (Is heart disease seen as an acute or chronic problem?)
- Causes
  (Changeable v unchangeable, e.g. family history or cigarette smoking)
- Consequences
  (Minor v major)
- Cure
  (Curable; chronic; terminal)

This model, the commonsense representation of illness model[14], has been shown to reflect the manner in which patients structure their views on a wide variety of illnesses.

A discussion on the understanding of heart disease can be usefully conducted at group level where patients can learn from the views of other patients. It is important to elicit the views of patients in group discussions rather than presenting the information in a didactic, classroom format. The former process is more engaging for patients and can help identify beliefs which may be unhelpful to the process of CR.

A recent study of the views of 50 Scottish MI patients[15] found common misconceptions about heart disease, including the following:

'Heart attack means the heart is worn out' (45% believe this)

'Pain with heart attack always means that more actual damage is being done' (60% believe this)

'Most people never return to previous levels of activity after a heart attack' (21% believe this)

'After a heart attack your sex life has to be modified forever' (13% believe this and another 27% are unsure)[1]. (see Note 1 at end of Chapter)

The issue of new and conflicting information, as presented in the media, e.g. on diet and heart disease, should be addressed with patients.

Overall, the knowledge component of the CR programme helps to agree a common agenda for professionals and patients. It also functions as an 'ice-breaker', helping patients in a group feel more comfortable talking about their views and concerns both among the group and in the presence of the CR professional.

Emotions management

Goals:
- An understanding of the range, function and impact of psychological reactions (emotions) experienced following a cardiac event;
- Recognition of these emotions as experienced by patients themselves;
- Identification of methods of managing emotions following cardiac events.

The widely used list of psychological reactions associated with stages of bereavement or reactions to the news of one's own terminal illness are useful since they focus on reactions to *loss* or impending loss. These stages are shock/denial, anger, bargaining, depression and acceptance. A coronary event may create a sense of loss – i.e. of one's former health, carefree life, capacity at work, in sexual relationship(s), in sporting or other roles. Thus many patients may feel far from 'lucky to be alive' following a coronary event. These emotions are considered in turn.

Denial

As mentioned earlier, denial is a common coping mechanism following an acute cardiac event. It ranges from complete denial of the event, to denial of the implications of the event – i.e. where patients 'deny' the possible negative implications of cardiac events, such as 'the meaning of life will never be the same', 'I will be permanently restricted', etc. – or it may have a protective effect on emotional well-being. Denial of the coronary event *per se* can result in either the performance of high risk behaviours, e.g. lifting or strenuous exercise without training or the continuation of previous unhealthy habits such as smoking and eating a high-fat diet.

A professional judgement of the role of denial for the patient may determine if particular aspects of denial should be directly challenged. Two questions can be usefully considered:

(1) Does 'denial' interfere with the recommendations of the CR programme?
   (If 'yes', then challenge the denial.)
(2) Does 'denial' serve a constructive function for the patient?
   (If 'yes', consider carefully before challenging and try to identify other supports, besides denial, for the patient.)

Anger

Patients, or relatives, may feel angry or hostile following a coronary event: 'Why me/us?', 'I've never smoked and have kept fit...', etc. Acknowledging a patient's anger, e.g. 'It must be very upsetting...', is usually a more useful response to such feelings than trying to explain or rationalize.

A range of patients are likely to show anger and hostility as part of a regular pre-coronary pattern of behaviour for them. This has been described as part of type A behaviour pattern (TABP), to be discussed more fully in the section on stress.

Bargaining

Many patients 'bargain' about medical treatments and lifestyle change: 'I'll do x if you guarantee to do y'. Bargaining may be with a spiritual being, fate, medical or other hospital staff. Thus patients sometimes want guarantees that their investment of energy and sacrifice in changing lifestyle will protect them against future cardiac events. CR staff must constantly emphasize the benefits of rehabilitation activities while at the same time emphasizing that *guarantees cannot be given* for specific patients or specific activities. In every instance, it should be emphasized that CR reduces the *probability* of recurrent events but *cannot be a guarantee* against them.

It is also important to have patients focus on short- or intermediate-term goals in CR. Thus, the objective need not – indeed should not – only be in significantly increasing longevity; rather, the focus should be on the ongoing enjoyment and quality of life to be had by following the advice as provided in CR programmes.

Anxiety

Anxiety is a state of apprehension, tension and worry which may be accompanied by physical symptoms such as rapid heart rate and respiration, sweating palms and dizziness[16]. For coronary patients, anxiety may be generalized, i.e. they feel anxious almost all of the time, or it may be specific (or worse) in particular situations such as taking exercise, attending the hospital, etc.

Typical symptoms of anxiety as experienced by CR participants are:

- Fear
- Agitation
- Heart palpitations
- Shaking or trembling
- Sweating
- Stomach churning ('butterflies in stomach')
- Difficulty concentrating
- Feeling helpless and out of control
- Inability to relax.

Anxiety is managed by:

- Teaching patients to relax (see later section on relaxation);
- Identifying the sources of anxiety of patients;
- Challenging either the cause or function of anxiety as experienced;
- Identifying the ABCs of experiences of anxiety;
- Learning how to reduce or avoid anxiety-arousing thoughts or situations.

Much of the purpose of CR is to reduce anxiety and to replace it with *self-efficacy* (Self-efficacy is described in greater detail in Chapter 5.). For instance, group exercise training on a CR programme helps participants to move (gradually) from a position of fearing any physical activity to calmly undertaking a significant weekly schedule of unsupervised exercise. It has been shown that routine cardiology procedures such as stress (treadmill) testing increases self-efficacy for patients[17] and that the self-efficacy increases following a CR programme[18].

Depression

Depression is a mood disorder whose main features are sadness and dejection, decreased motivation, decreased interest in life, negative thoughts (e.g. feeling hopeless or low in self-esteem) and physical symptoms (e.g. disturbed sleep, chronic fatigue and loss of appetite and energy[16]) Depression is one of the most common emotions experienced by patients in the period after an acute cardiac event. Cardiac patients also report higher levels of depression before medical events than is usual in similar community groups. Thus in managing depression in CR, it is important to establish how long the patient has been feeling this way. Significant levels of pre-existing depression may not resolve with brief, usually group, CR intervention and onward referral strategies should be in place as discussed later. It is also important to consider that depression is associated with drop-out from CR programmes[19], thus significant early efforts to manage depression in a CR group are important.

Typical symptoms of depression as experienced by CR participants are:

- Sadness
- Lack of interest in events
- Inability to experience joy or pleasure
- Feelings of inadequacy and self-blame
- Negative view of the world and of the future
- Difficulty concentrating
- Feeling that life is not worth living
- Feeling tearful
- Inability to initiate activities
- Loss of affection and concern for others
- Sleep disturbance
- Fatigue and lack of energy
- Loss of appetite and sexual interest.

People who are depressed often have three components to their negative thinking; the problem is:

- Internal (v external): 'It's my fault.'
- Stable (v changeable): 'It will always be like this'
- Global (v specific): 'It will affect my whole life'.

Depression is managed by having individuals:

- Identify the negative thoughts they engage in;
- Challenge those negative perceptions;
- Identify the ABCs of these perceptions (see later the ABC of behaviour);
- Learn how to reduce negative thoughts and substitute with positive statements;
- Increase the experience of positive events including social interaction;
- Increase assertiveness.

A number of specific emotions have been described to date. A major component of CR programmes is the management of stress. Stress is an umbrella term which may include the experience and management of a range of emotions outlined above.

Stress

Stress is sometimes seen as a *response* to external situations ('having a heart attack causes stress') or as a *stimulus* or initiator of external situations ('stress causes a heart attack'). More usefully, stress is seen as an *interaction* between person and environment where the individual *perceives* that that the demands being placed on him or her exceed the available resources and therefore threaten his or her well-being[16]. The *perception* that demands are beyond the individual's capabilities may be accurate or inaccurate but the important point in stress is that they are perceived to be so. This is the key to stress management. Stress management is about coping with the stressor in an appropriate manner.

Coping

Coping is the process by which individuals manage stressful situations[16]. Two forms of coping are possible: *problem-focused* coping, where individuals try to cope with stress directly by changing or avoiding circumstances, and *emotion-focused* coping, where individuals cope indirectly by managing the emotions surrounding the stressful experience.

Problem-focused coping:
- Change situation
    environment (e.g. move to less stressful job)
    self (e.g. lower personal aspirations)
- Avoid situation
    (e.g. cancel scheduled course or appointment)

Emotion-focused coping:
- Cognitive: i.e. change thoughts
    (e.g. seeing positive aspects of illness)
- Behavioural: i.e. change behaviour
    (e.g. taking exercise to relax).

Neither type of coping is always helpful or unhelpful. For instance, using exercise is an emotion-focused coping strategy, but so too is drinking alcohol. Particular individuals may have a general style of coping which is not always appropriate. Thus problem-focused coping is not always an appropriate response for primarily emotional difficulties and emotion-focused coping, e.g. over-eating or over-drinking, is not an appropriate stress management technique – especially for cardiac patients.

When CR participants display a range of unusual activities it is useful to think of these as coping strategies and consider what purpose they serve for the individual. A basis for good stress management is being able to practise relaxation as a coping strategy.

Relaxation

If individuals have been stressed over a period of time, they are often not even aware of their stress or their inability to relax. Thus a first challenge in stress management may be to have individuals make a realistic assessment of their level of tension. There can also be a feeling that relaxation is easy and involves simply 'doing nothing' or, conversely, that it involves strange exercises or activities which CR participants may feel wary or shy about adopting. Subsequent attitudes to stress management may depend on the style in which they are introduced. It is important to de-mystify the techniques and present them as practical, coping strategies.

Methods of relaxation are numerous and variable. Most involve the individual selecting a comfortable sitting or reclining position. A quiet peaceful environment, often with the light subdued, is ideal. Otherwise the individual may become distracted and have difficulty concentrating or relaxing. Most methods of relaxation help focus attention on various parts of the body and then relaxing the muscles in that area. The relaxation training which is most widely recommended consists of the individual practising tensing and releasing muscle groups in turn until he or she is able to relax and concentrate on the corresponding sensations with the minimum of prompting.

Unfortunately, some individuals can become anxious and develop panic attacks during progressive muscle relaxation. Thus it is advisable to ensure that the individual breathes normally during relaxation and is warned against holding the breath during some exercises and then taking deep gasps to recover – which may amount to hyperventilation.

Relaxation training should be taught as an active coping technique for use in real-life situations. Initially, it will be taught by an instructor whilst the participant is lying down or sitting in a well-supported position, but soon after the technique should be self-applied, usually by the self-administration of an audio-cassette tape. The latter offers a low cost, readily available method of tension and anxiety reduction. Where relaxation tapes are provided to participants, it may be more beneficial to have the tape narrated by a member of the CR programme staff than to offer a commercial tape of unfamiliar origin.

Learning to use relaxation skills is best achieved using three interacting approaches[20]:

- Learning relaxation skills;
- Learning to identify and monitor tension in daily life;
- Learning to use relaxation skills at times of stress.

Skills development and maintenance

Goals:
- Development of a range of health behaviours with professional advice on appropriate methods and targets;
- Development of strategies for maintaining health behaviours over time and outside the physical location of the CR programme.

A helpful framework in this regard is the ABC framework described next.

ABC of behaviour and behaviour change

It is useful to consider behaviour, whether negative (e.g. over-eating) or positive (e.g. taking moderate exercise), using the ABC framework[21].

'A' relates to the **antecedents**, or factors predicting a target behaviour
'B' is the target **behaviour**
'C' are the **consequences** of the target behaviour.

In the model shown in Table 6.1, a more positive outcome could be promoted by encouraging a change in antecedents – for example, for an individual living alone to arrange for callers or to go out more socially. This could avoid the danger of bingeing on food additional to requirements. Most lifestyle-associated behaviours are performed because of memories of positive consequences of these behaviours on previous occasions. The challenge in CR is to associate healthy lifestyle activities such as exercising and eating low-fat foods with positive memories.

Table 6.1   Influence on the performance of healthy or risky behaviours: the ABC framework. (Adapted from Russell[21], p. 20.)

Antecedents (examples)	Behaviour (examples)	Consequences (examples)
External situation Living alone.		
		External situation Becoming overweight.
Thoughts and feelings Lonely and depressed.	**Healthy or risky behaviour** Eating outside of mealtimes.	
		Thoughts and feelings Immediate consolation; guilt later.
Behaviour Watching TV.		

Perceived outcome of various behaviours

Unhealthy behaviours

- Immediate consequences are positive, e.g. taste of high-fat food;
- Long-term consequences are negative, e.g. cigarette smoking increases health risk.

Healthy behaviours

- Immediate consequences are negative, e.g. feel stiff after exercising;
- Long-term consequences are positive, e.g. weight reduction results in increased energy and self-esteem.

The role of CR is to support participants by educating them about the negative long-term consequences of unhealthy behaviours and by giving them sufficient experience of healthy behaviours so that they start to identify some longer-term consequences of their activities. In time and with practice, it is also expected that many of the immediate consequences of healthy behaviours, e.g. the taste of healthier foods and the sensation of exercising, will be experienced as positive in themselves.

Type A behaviour pattern

One particular pattern of behaviour frequently associated with cardiac patients is type A behaviour pattern (TABP). This is a style of behaviour associated with being:

- Rushed, speedy, and always short of time;
- Competitive, driven and extremely achievement oriented;
- Impatient, aggressive and hostile.

This pattern was initially described by two cardiologists, Friedman and Rosenman, over 30 years ago. They felt it typified their coronary patients. While a large volume of early evidence suggested that people who were type A as distinct from type B (not showing the above characteristics) were at higher risk for developing heart disease, more recent evidence has failed to find a negative health effect of TABP. Instead, research has focused on the three components of TABP as outlined above and hostility has emerged as the behaviour pattern most associated with risk of heart disease[22].

Several interventions have, to varying degrees, been successful in modifying TABP, including exercise and cognitive-behavioural therapy. Combinations of treatment techniques appear to be most effective. An assessment involves individuals identifying what triggers TABP and how they respond to it[20]. Strategies to change can then be developed. The management of TABP is probably best accomplished by the participant attending a course of small-group meetings, lasting about one hour, which include:

- Education on the nature of TABP and its potential association with coronary disease;
- Self-appraisal of cognitions and cognitive restructuring;
- Anxiety management;

- Anger control (including assertiveness training);
- Relaxation techniques.

Each session should allow participants to provide examples of the subject being discussed and a pooling of coping styles and resources, and end with a period of relaxation. Between sessions, behavioural objectives should be set, and a diary of responses kept. Measures of TABP, hostility, anger and anxiety should be taken during the initial assessment and subsequently before and after treatment.

Role restoration

A final target of psychosocial intervention is the restoration of previous core roles for the patient. The two most commonly focused on in CR programmes are the restoration of sexual activities following a coronary event, and the return to vocational role functioning. Many patients experience serious role disruption following a cardiac event. Often the threat or belief that a particularly valued role, e.g. sexual partner or competent employee, can no longer be maintained is a major source of distress for patients.

Goals:
- To restore patient to previous levels of participation in a range of social roles where appropriate (i.e. health promoting) and achievable (i.e. clinically advisable);
- To support the changes required to achieve an acceptable level of role functioning in domains where complete role restoration is not possible (e.g. job restructuring in a physically demanding environment).

Sexual activity

Many people, and their partners, experience lack of interest in or fear of sexual activities following a major coronary event[23]. Failure of the CR professional to discuss the topic may contribute to sexual dysfunction. Sexual concerns and anxiety should be addressed early and sexual counselling should be part of early CR. Partners should be included in such counselling wherever possible.

Some individuals, particularly the elderly, will find it extremely difficult to talk about sex and the CR professional should help by initiating the discussion. Individuals should be given information about the resumption of sexual activity and invited to discuss any fears or concerns that they have.

It is likely that sexual difficulties are largely attributable to psychological factors compounded by inadequate information. Participants need to be assured that sexual activity is not a major problem in terms of increased risk of cardiac morbidity or mortality. The provision of printed material, auditory or visual tapes should be supplemented with further explanation and question answering to assure comprehension and avoid misinterpretations.

The P-LI-SS-IT model[24] provides a useful four-level framework for those involved in dealing with the sexual concerns of CR participants:

(1) **P (Permission):** Giving permission to discuss and ask questions about sex – for example: 'Many people are worried about when they can resume sex. I wonder whether there are any questions or concerns that you or your partner have regarding your sexual relationship?'
(2) **LI (Limited Information):** The need to provide a couple with factual information directly relevant to their particular situation and sexual concerns – depending on the individual's sex, age, physical condition and expectations. For example, the fact that after a cardiac event, sexual activity should be resumed gradually and carefully – in the same way as other types of physical activity. General advice would include the avoidance of sex with an unfamiliar partner, after a heavy meal, when intoxicated, or when fatigued.
(3) **SS (Specific Suggestions):** These will depend on the problem. Careful and detailed assessment of the individual's problem, goals and expectation is necessary. Specific suggestions vary, but are generally aimed at reducing anxiety associated with sex and at facilitating communication between the couple. If the sexual problem remains unresolved, it may be necessary to proceed to the fourth level of intervention.
(4) **IT (Intensive Therapy):** Referral to a sexual counsellor or clinical psychologist. Sometimes a sexual dysfunction clinic appointment may be indicated.

Vocational rehabilitation

Return to work has traditionally been used as a broad indicator of restoration of functioning following a serious coronary event. This may involve return to paid employment outside the family home and/or the regular duties undertaken by the individual before the onset of health problems. While some activities and occupations need to be appraised for safety in terms of their physiological workload, in many situations it will be more important to promote the confidence of the CR participant in the psychological challenge to return to former activities. Where individuals have the option either to continue in an employment situation or to retire, it is useful to advise caution in making hasty decisions: serious and life-long decisions may be better made at some distance in time from the cardiac event and after the opportunity to complete the CR programme. Some CR participants will require assistance in appraising the advisability of returning to their prior work requirements. Work environments may be excessively demanding because of their psychological or physical requirements. For the former, instruction on stress management, including time management, is appropriate.

A very simple rule of thumb regarding time management is one-third sleep, one-third work and one-third social and leisure activities. Where physical requirements are excessive for cardiac patients, the advice of a vocational officer may be important in planning for retraining or in facilitating redeployment at the individual's workplace. In some circumstances, a vocational officer can assist in allaying the anxieties of an employer about having an employee with cardiac problems return to the workplace[25].

General difficulties

A range of other difficulties may arise from time to time with CR participants. There may be difficulties associated with a particular type of cardiac event, for instance, post-operative delirium is sometimes experienced by bypass or open-heart surgery patients[26] and may need specific intervention with patient and/or family to manage anxieties following the episode. Similarly, neuropsychological difficulties, typically presenting as difficulty with concentration, remembering or retrieving information, may be associated with bypass patients[27]. It is not clear in research studies if these problems usually predate surgery or are a result of the bypass procedure. From the CR perspective, the implication is the same – management of the presenting problem. An important consideration here is whether concentration difficulties are diminished alongside reduction in depression or anxiety for patients. In a small number of cases, where concentration difficulties continue to be significant, onward referral for neuropsychological assessment is warranted.

A general point about a range of miscellaneous problems which arise in the psychosocial area is to maintain a clear perspective on what should be the brief of a CR programme and what should be referred elsewhere – for example on-going sexual difficulties, problems with alcohol or other substance abuse, neuropsychological difficulties, vocational worries, psychiatric difficulties, etc., are all outside the CR remit and necessitate proper referral. Many of the difficulties experienced by patients may be experienced in their interaction with others, e.g. with an anxious or overprotective or unsupportive partner. As with achieving target behaviours regarding exercise and diet, it is important to address the specific concerns of close family members in the CR programme[28]. Many programmes include partners at one or more time-points in their schedule.

In a small number of cases, significant psychological problems may pre-date the presentation of cardiac disease. These cases represent a particular challenge as such patients may feel that the motivation required to participate in structured CR programmes is beyond their capabilities. Depending on the nature of the problems, the assistance of qualified mental health professionals, including the option of referral of the patient to the services of relevance to the patient's problem(s) (e.g. addiction services) should be considered. These patients can be considered for CR services in tandem with such support or following completion of other forms of therapy as appropriate.

Psychosocial service delivery

Psychosocial services to a CR programme should be provided by a staff member with mental health training. In some settings it is possible to have a qualified mental health practitioner (e.g. psychologist, psychiatrist, nurse or counsellor) provide all of the CR programme input and this is ideal both for input and continuity. In other settings, general information provision and explanation regarding psychological reactions following a coronary event may be provided by any other health professional. It is, however, to be recommended strongly that a number of psychosocial sessions with CR groups are conducted by a qualified mental health professional or other health professional who has undergone specific counselling training. This is to ensure both the standard of general delivery of psychosocial care to CR participants and that particular and more occasional difficulties, e.g. subtle neuropsychological problems, are identified and appropriately managed.

Liaison with the mental health section of the hospital may facilitate both service provision to the CR programme and the transfer of particular difficulties to specialist care. It is also important in a CR programme that both the skills and the responsibility for managing all aspects of lifestyle are transferred in a supportive but clear manner from the CR professional to the participant. Mental health professionals can assist other staff in developing self-management strategies and in providing an overall service which assists participants to transfer the skills learned in CR to their lives in general.

Outcomes of psychosocial interventions

It is important to measure the psychosocial outcome of patients following CR in order to demonstrate improvement in, or maintenance of, good psychosocial functioning. Many instruments are potentially available to measure aspects of psychosocial functioning, but as yet the evidence has not been collected to identify the definitive set of brief measures to capture the psychosocial needs of cardiac patients and the impact of the CR programme on these needs. A number of measures which have been used are described here. Traditionally, specific individual topics, such as depression or anxiety, have been evaluated, while more recently quality-of-life has been discussed as an 'umbrella' concept covering a range of aspects of psychosocial well-being including social, emotional, cognitive and vocational functioning.

Quality of life

Quality of life is a widely used concept in current health care[29]. Its range of usage as a term includes:

■ A description of health economic evaluations within or across services;
■ Professional assessments of the performance of patients on a number of clinically relevant measures;
■ Individuals' own assessments of how much their collective set of circumstances – including health, psychological, social and vocational functioning – add up to a satisfying, or otherwise, life.

In the context of assessing a CR programme, the latter objective of evaluating the individual's perspective is the appropriate focus of evaluation. 'Quality-of-life' encompasses a broad range of physical and psychological characteristics and limitations which describe an individual's ability to function and to derive satisfaction from doing so. In its simplest form, a patient's quality of life is what he or she says it is, since subjective evaluation is essential to quality-of-life assessment. In this regard, the patient's perspective, rather than the values or the views of the CR professional, becomes the important consideration in quality of life evaluations. Quality-of-life is an important concept in CR since it combines the negative and positive aspects of the participant's overall experience of living with and managing coronary disease. It is also a useful focus to keep in mind as a CR professional, since many of the activities encouraged need to be experienced by participants as contributing significantly to their quality of life – as well as to their likely quantity of life if they are to be maintained in the longer term. Discussion of a number of instruments to measure quality of life is outlined in the next section.

Instruments to assess psychosocial function

Psychosocial instruments complement measures of functional status in providing an overall picture of patient status before and after a CR programme. It is important to emphasize that there is as yet no agreement on the ideal set of instruments to assess psychosocial functioning. Practical considerations for patients, such as the length, comprehensibility and acceptability of the instrument, should be considered: Do your patients find it too lengthy, too difficult to understand, or comprising of questions which are seen as too embarrassing or too sensitive to answer? The only method of addressing these queries is to try the instrument you have selected on a small but mixed group of patients. In order to be able to compare your findings with those at other centres, it is essential that you include all questions from the original instruments and in the original format so that standard scoring systems may apply. Practical considerations for the CR professional must also be taken into account. Is the measure easily and speedily scorable? Can the findings be easily interpreted as being clinically meaningful, e.g. what score ranges on a depression scale depict mild, moderate or severe depression?

Two further points of concern in choosing instruments to measure psychosocial function in CR participants are that they should focus on the less severe end of the spectrum since for most people there will not be evidence of severe psychopathology; also they should be measures which are sensitive to change in this population. On the latter point, instruments which document most participants as being at the better extreme of psychosocial functioning before CR may be insensitive because of the 'ceiling' effect – i.e. it is difficult to show whether participants improve over time because most have already reached their maximum score. Similarly, with measures of extreme psychosocial difficulties, it may be that as very few participants report these problems at the outset (the 'floor' effect), it becomes difficult to illustrate the benefits of the CR programme on general psychosocial functioning.

The instruments outlined next represent only a small selection of those currently available. They have been chosen primarily because they are relatively brief (thus improving the likelihood that they can be used as routine assessment tools rather than simply as research instruments) and because they have already been used with cardiac patients. References are to studies which have used these instruments with a cardiac population. From these references, more detailed lists of references, including sources for the original instruments, can be obtained.

Anxiety

Hospital Anxiety and Depression (HAD) Scale: This is a 14-item measure with seven items each for anxiety and depression. Questions are rated on a 4-point subscale from 'No problems' to 'Significant problems'. A cut-off point for each subscale allows identification of those high in anxiety or depression or both. The measure is widely used in a range of medical populations and is popular because of its brevity and acceptability to patients[30].

State-Trait Anxiety Inventory (STAI): This measures general (trait) and situation-specific (state) anxiety. Each section comprises 20 items. In repeat measurements, the trait questions need not be re-completed by patients as, by definition, trait anxiety does not change over time. The measure has been widely used in medical, including cardiology, populations[31,32].

Depression

Hospital Anxiety and Depression (HAD) Scale: See previous section.

Zung Self-Rating Depression Scale: This is a 20-item scale with each question having a 4-point grading from low degree of impairment to high degree of impairment[33].

Quality of life

Nottingham Health Profile (NHP): This is a two-part questionnaire measuring a range of aspects of quality of life. Part I has 38 questions to assess the degree of discomfort or distress experienced by individuals on six dimensions: energy, sleep, pain, emotional reaction, mobility and social isolation. Scores range from no problems to problems on every aspect of the dimension queried. Part II comprises 7 Yes/No questions assessing the occurrence of health-related problems with regard to paid employment, housework, hobbies, family life, sex life, social life and holidays. General community figures are available by age and sex for the NHP in the UK: these provide useful comparison opportunities with CR groups[34,35]. As a very widely used scale, many other comparisons are available with a variety of patient groups and interventions. On the other hand, the NHP provides a profile of patient scores across such areas as pain, sleep and energy which cannot be summarized to form an overall score. This can make pre-CR and post-CR comparisons difficult if some aspects of quality of life improve and others diminish over time for patients. This measure should be used only after consultation with its authors.

Quality of Life after Myocardial Infarction Questionnaire: This is a recently developed 26-item measure comprising 5 factors grouped into two dimensions: limitations (including symptoms and restrictions) and emotions (including emotional function, confidence and self-esteem). It has been used in a CR study where patients randomly assigned to a CR programme were shown to improve in quality of life more rapidly than matched patients[36]. Differences between the groups converged and at one year post-MI, a higher but similar quality of life was evident in both groups.

Short Form-36 (SF-36): This is a 36-item questionnaire derived from a large scale research project called the Medical Outcomes Study. It covers eight aspects of health-related quality of life: physical functioning, mental health, general health perception, physical role limitation, emotional role functioning, social functioning, bodily pain and vitality. It is being widely used in a range of medical populations in the UK and elsewhere[37] and two large regional samples (Sheffield and Oxford) provide general population data on patterns of scoring[38]. Evaluation of a CR sample (N = 157) before and after a 12-week programme showed significant improvement on all sub-scales[39]. A larger study (N = 789) has evaluated participants at the start of a CR programme and compared performance with community samples[40]. Cardiac patients were most impaired in physical functioning and vitality. Follow-up data on this group is being collected.

Mood

Profile of Mood States (POMS): This is a 65-adjective scale assessing six aspects of mood: tension–anxiety, depression–rejection, anger–hostility, vigour, fatigue and confusion–bewilderment. Each adjective represents a feeling that is rated from 'Not experienced at all' to 'Extreme experience'[41].

Summary of key points

- A range of psychosocial issues can and should be addressed in the CR setting.
- An explicit focus on managing psychosocial concerns can increase both the cardiac patient's quality of life and his or her management of a health-promoting lifestyle.
- Good psychosocial outcome should not be expected as a by-product of cardiovascular (exercise) rehabilitation but rather planned for and included as a specific aspect of multidisciplinary rehabilitation following a cardiac event.

References

1. Smith, T.W. and Leon, A.S. (1992) *Coronary Heart Disease: A Behavioral Perspective*, Champaign, Illinois: Research Press.
   [A general overview of psychosocial factors in both the development of heart disease and in the management of coronary events.]
2. Amarosa-Tupler, B., Tapp, J.T. and Carida, R.V. (1989) Stress management through relaxation and imagery in the treatment of angina pectoris, *Journal of Cardiopulmonary Rehabilitation*, **9**, 348–55.
3. Bundy, C., Carroll, D., Wallace, L. and Nagle, R. (1994) Psychological treatment of chronic stable angina pectoris, *Psychology and Health*, **10**, 69–77.
4. Lewin, B., Robertson, I.H., Cay, E.L., Irving, J.B. and Campbell, M. (1992) Effects of self-help post-myocardial infarction rehabilitation on psychological adjustment and use of health services, *Lancet*, **329**, 1036–40.
5. Schockern, D.D., Green, D.F., Worden, T. J., Hamison, E.E. and Spielberger, C.D. (1987) Effects of age on the relationship between anxiety and coronary artery disease, *Psychosomatic Medicine*, **49**, 118–26.
6. Schleifer, S. J., Macari-Hinson, M.M., Coyle, D.A., Slater, W.R., Kahn, M., Gorlin, R. and Zucker, H.D. (1989) The nature and course of depression following myocardial infarction, *Archives of Internal Medicine*, **149**, 1785–9.
7. Frasure-Smith, N., Lesperance, F. and Talajic, M. (1993) Depression following myocardial infarction: Impact on 6-month survival, *Journal of the American Medical Association*, **270**, 1819–25.
8. Coyne, J.C. and Smith, D.A.F. (1991) Couples coping with a myocardial infarction: a contextual perspective on wives' distress, *Journal of Personality and Social Psychology*, **61**, 404–12.
9. Van Dixhoorn, J., Diuvenvoorden, H.J., Staal, H.A. and Pool, J. (1989) Physical training and relaxation therapy in cardiac rehabilitation assessed

through a composite criterion for training outcome, *American Heart Journal*, **118**, 545–52.

10. Leon, S., Certo, C., Comoss, P. *et al.* (1990) Position paper of the American Association of Cardiovascular and Pulmonary Rehabilitation. Scientific evidence of the value of cardiac rehabilitation services with emphasis on patients following myocardial infarction – Section I: exercise conditioning component. *Journal of Cardiopulmonary Rehabilitation*, **10**, 79–87.

11. McGee, H.M. (1995) Can the measurement of quality of life contribute to evaluation in cardiac rehabilitation services? *Journal of Cardiovascular Risk* 2,(in press).

12. Anda, R.F., Williamson, D.F., Escobedo, L.G., Mast, E.E., Giovino, G.A. and Remington, P.L. (1990) Depression and the dynamics of smoking, *Journal of the American Medical Association*, **264**, 1541–5.

13. Ley, P. (1992) *Communicating with Patients*, London: Croom Helm.

14. Leventhal, H., Meyer, D., Nerenz, D. (1980) The common-sense representation of illness danger. In S. Rachman (ed.), *Medical Psychology* Vol II, New York: Pergamon Press, pp. 7–30.

15. Foulkes, J. (1994) *Cardiac Rehabilitation in the Acute Post-Myocardial Infarction Period.* Master of Philosophy Thesis, University of St Andrews, Scotland. [See also Foulkes, J., Johnston, M., Robertson, C. (1993) Knowledge and distress: implications of cardiac recovery programmes. In J. Wilson-Barnett and J. MacLeod-Clark (eds.), *Health Promotion and Nursing Research*, London: Macmillan, pp. 197–203.]

16. Atkinson, R.L., Atkinson, R.C., Smith, E.E., Bem, D.J. and Hilgard, E.R. (1990) *Introduction to Psychology*, New York: Harcourt Brace Jovanovich. [A general text with useful outline of stress coping, anxiety and depression.]

17. Ewart, C.K., Taylor, C.B., Reese, L.B. and DeBusk, R.F. (1983) Effects of early postmyocardial infarction exercise testing on self-perceptions and subsequent physical activity, *American Journal of Cardiology*, **51**, 1076–80. [A subsequent study by the same research group showed that having a spouse witness the performance of the patient on exercise testing increased the confidence of the spouse in the patient's abilities: Taylor, C.B., Bandura, A., Ewart, C.K., Miller, N.H. and DeBusk, R.F. (1985) Exercise testing to enhance wives' confidence in their husband's cardiac capacity soon after a clinically uncomplicated myocardial infarction, *American Journal of Cardiology*, **55**, 635–8.]

18. McGee, H.M. and Horgan, J.H. (1995) Patient self-efficacy and quality of life following cardiac rehabilitation (submitted for publication).

19. Blumenthal, J.A., Williams, R.S., Wallace, A.G., Williams, R.B. and Needles, T.L. (1982) Physiological and psychological variables predict compliance to prescribed exercise therapy in patients recovering from myocardial infarction, *Psychosomatic Medicine*, **44**, 519–27.

20. Bennett, P. (1993) *Counselling for Heart Disease*, Leicester: British Psychological Society Books.

[Useful text outlining psychosocial concerns of cardiac patients.]

21. Russell, M.R. (1986) *Behavioral Counselling in Medicine*, New York: Oxford University Press.

22. McGee, H.M., Graham, T. and Horgan, J.H. (1994) Heart Disease: the Psychological Challenge. *Irish Journal of Psychology* **15**, (1).
[Special issue of the journal with two papers addressing type A behaviour pattern and others assessing quality of life and neuropsychological difficulties.]

23. Papadopoulos, C. (1992) Sexual problems/interventions. In N.K. Wenger and H.K. Hellerstein (eds.), *Rehabilitation of the Coronary Patient*, New York: Churchill Livingstone, pp. 473–81.

24. Annon, J.S. (1976) *The Behavioural Treatment of Sexual Problems: Brief Therapy*, New York: Harper & Row.

25. Massey, M.A. (1994) Involving State vocational counsellors in serving cardiopulmonary program participants, *Journal of Cardiopulmonary Rehabilitation*, **14**, 25–6.

26. Prochaska, J.O. and DiClemente, C.C. (1992) Stages of change in the modification of problem behaviours. In M. Hersen, R.M. Eisler and P.M. Miller (eds), *Progress in Behaviour Modification*, Sycamore: Sycamore Press, pp. 183–219.

27. Shaw, P.J., Bates, D., Cartilage, N.E.F. *et al.* (1989) An analysis of factors predisposing to neurological injury in patients undergoing coronary bypass operations, *Quarterly Journal of Medicine*, **267**, 633–46.

28. McGee, H.M., Graham, T., Newton, H. and Horgan, J.H. (1994) The involvement of the spouse in cardiac rehabilitation, *Irish Journal of Psychology*, **15**, 203–18.

29. Mayou, R. and Bryant, B. (1993) Quality of life in cardiovascular disease, *British Heart Journal*, **69**, 460–6.
[Useful outline of general issues to consider when choosing a quality of life instrument)

30. Zigmond, A.S. and Snaith, R.P. (1983) The Hospital Anxiety and Depression Scale. *Acta Psychiatrica Scandinavica*, **67**, 361–70.

31. Jenkins, C.D., Stanton, B.A., Savageau, J.A., Denlinger, P. and Klein, M.D. (1983) Coronary artery bypass surgery: Physical, psychological, social and economic outcomes six months later, *Journal of the American Medical Association*, **250**, 782–3.
[Used Spielberger State-Trait Anxiety Inventory]

32. Rovario, S., Holmes, D.S. and Holmsten, R.D. (1984) Influence of a cardiac rehabilitation programme on the cardiovascular, psychological and social functioning of cardiac patients, *Journal of Behavioural Medicine*, **7**, 61–81.
[Used Spielberger State-Trait Anxiety Inventory and Beck Depression Inventory.]

33. Taylor, C.B., DeBusk, R.F., Davidson, D.M., Houston, N. and Burnett, K. (1981) Optimal methods of identifying depression following hospitalisation

for myocardial infarction, *Journal of Chronic Diseases*, **34**, 127–33.
[Used Zung Self-Rating Scale for Depression.]

34. Wiklund, I., Herlitz, J. and Hjalmarson, A. (1989) Quality of life five years after myocardial infarction, *European Heart Journal*, **10**, 464–72.
[Used Nottingham Health Profile.]

35. O'Brien, B.J., Buxton, M.J. and Ferguson, B.A. (1987) Measuring the effectiveness of heart transplant programmes: quality of life data and their relationship to survival analysis, *Journal of Chronic Diseases*, **40** (suppl. 1) 137S–53S.

36. Oldridge, N., Guyatt, G., Jones, N., Crowe, J. and Singer, J. (1991) Effects on quality of life with comprehensive rehabilitation after acute myocardial infarction, *American Journal of Cardiology*, **67**, 1084–9.
[Used Quality of Life after Myocardial Infarction Questionnaire.]

37. Spertus, J.A., Winder, J.A., Dewhurst, T.A., Deyo, R.A. and Fihn, S.D. (1994) Monitoring the quality of life in patients with coronary artery disease, *American Journal of Cardiology*, **74**, 1240–4.
[Used SF-36.]

38. Jenkinson, C., Wright, L. and Coulter, A. (*1993*) *Quality of Life Measurement in Health Care. A Review of Measures and Population norms for the UK SF-36*, University of Oxford: Health Services Research Unit.

39. Lavie, C.J. and Milani, R.V. (1995) Effects of cardiac rehabilitation and exercise training on exercise capacity, coronary risk factors, behavioural characteristics and quality of life in women. *American Journal of Cardiology*, **75**, 340–3.

40. Jette, D.V. and Dowling, J. (1994) Health Status of individuals entering a cardiac rehabilitation program as measured by the Medical Outcomes Study 36-item short form survey (SF-36). *Physical Therapy*, **74**, 521–7.

41. Kemkes, B.M., Augerman, C.E. and Bullinger, M. (1991) Quality of life assessment in heart transplanation, *Theoretical Surgery*, **6**, 195–200.
[Used Profile of Mood States.]

Notes

Note 1. A 19-item Knowledge Questionnaire eliciting beliefs and misconceptions was developed for this study. Each item is rated as Correct, Incorrect (a misconception), or 'Don't know' (uncertain). A copy of the scale is available from Professor Marie Johnston, School of Psychology, University of St Andrew's, Fife, Scotland KY16 9JU.

Chapter 7

Dietary Aspects of Cardiac Rehabilitation

Summary

There is a consistent body of evidence linking diet with cardiovascular disease. Diet influences cardiovascular disease through its effect on some of the risk factors for coronary heart disease (CHD), mainly high cholesterol and blood pressure and to a lesser extent obesity, diabetes mellitus and thrombogenic factors. This chapter discusses aspects of diet and CHD and their relevance to cardiac rehabilitation, including modifiable dietary risk factors and cholesterol levels.

Modifiable risk factors

Diet is an important modifiable risk factor in the of management of cardiovascular disease,[1] and is of paramount importance in both primary and secondary prevention of the disease. The cardioprotective diet is an essential part of a cardiac rehabilitation (CR) programme and eating for a healthy heart should be seen as a positive and enjoyable lifestyle change.

Evidence exists of overall benefit in secondary prevention studies of lowering blood cholesterol and thereby decreasing CHD morbidity and mortality. There is a positive association between serum cholesterol and CHD, and serum cholesterol levels can be reduced by dietary modification. A lipid-lowering diet can reduce blood cholesterol by 10–20% and even more if accompanied by weight loss. A decrease in serum cholesterol of 1% represents a 2% decrease in CHD risk[2].

The British Hyperlipidaemia Association (BHA) has stated that hypercholesterolaemia should not be treated on the basis of a numerical value of the cholesterol level only, but by an assessment of the overall cardiovascular risk of the individual patient[3]. Priority is given to patients with established CHD including myocardial infarction (MI), post-coronary artery bypass grafting (CABG), angioplasty, cardiac transplant, or with other significant atherosclerosis. The

BHA recommends vigorous cholesterol lowering therapy to be introduced in this high risk group, i.e. patients with the following levels:

- Total cholesterol above 5.2 mmols/l
- Low density lipoprotein (LDL) cholesterol above 3.4 mmols/l
- High density lipoprotein (HDL) cholesterol below 1.0 mmols/l
- Triglycerides above 2.3 mmols/l.

If one considers that 60% of the adult population have serum cholesterol levels above 5.2 mmols/l, then it is logical that most CR patients will need some cholesterol-lowering advice. Very high cholesterol levels (over 8 mmols/l) are seen in patients with familial hypercholesterolaemia (about 1 in 500 of the general population). These patients should be referred to a lipid clinic and family lipid screening organized.

Therapeutic goals

The goals to aim for in patients with established CHD or other significant atherosclerosis are:

- Total cholesterol below 5.2 mmols/l
- LDL cholesterol below 3.4 mmols/l.

Low density lipoprotein (LDL) transports cholesterol from the liver to the cells in the body, including the atherosclerotic plaques. LDL cholesterol levels can be calculated using the Friedwald equation:

$$\text{LDL chol} = \text{Total cholesterol} - \text{HDL cholesterol} - \text{triglycerides} \div 2.19$$
(applicable when total triglyceride levels are less than 4.5 mmols/l)

HDL scavenges excess cholesterol and transports it from the tissues back to the liver, including from the atherosclerotic plaques, for eventual excretion. Higher levels of LDL cholesterol are associated with greater risk of CHD. Higher levels of HDL cholesterol (which acts as an arterial 'hoover') are associated with lower risks of CHD.

Triglycerides act as an independent risk factor for CHD, particularly when accompanied by a low HDL cholesterol[4]. Mild hypertriglyceridaemia (3–6 mmols/l) is often seen in obese people, those with diabetes and those who abuse alcohol. Higher concentrations of triglycerides, over 6 mmols/l, are associated with a risk of pancreatitis.

The first line treatment of an elevated lipid profile is dietary advice. However, if after an adequate time (at least three to six months) on a lipid-lowering diet, the profile has not modified sufficiently, appropriate drug treatment may need to be initiated with continued diet therapy.

For CR patients, lipid profiles should always include HDL cholesterol for more specific risk assessment and the sample should be taken fasting (16 hours) for an accurate triglyceride result. The first profile should be taken during the first 24 hours after an MI or six to twelve weeks later to obtain an accurate result. Any physical trauma, including cardiac events such as MI and CABG, has the effect of reducing serum cholesterol concentrations and elevating triglyceride levels.

Diet and hypertension

Epidemiologically, countries with high rates of hypertension have high salt intakes. Sodium intake appears to be an important determinant of blood pressure in the population as a whole or partly by influencing the rise of blood pressure with age[5]. The present intake of sodium in the diet from common salt exceeds that required to meet metabolic needs. Conversely, potassium from fruit and vegetables in the diet can help reduce blood pressure, and the ratio of sodium-to-potassium-containing foods in the diet may be more important then the sodium content of the diet alone. Alcohol intake and obesity are also thought to influence blood pressure. Binge drinking is particularly hazardous for increased risk of stroke and death. Raised blood pressure can be reduced by normalizing weight, reducing salt intake, increasing potassium intake from fruit and vegetables and limiting alcohol.

Diet and excess weight

Being overweight, i.e. having a body mass index (BMI: see Appendix 6) of 25–30, and obesity (BMI of 30 plus) are not independent risk factors for CHD but are associated with hyperlipidaemia, hypertension and high insulin levels. Being overweight results from a surplus intake of energy over energy expended, which is stored as fat. Despite the adult population trends to decrease calorie and fat intake, Britons are still getting fatter as not enough energy is being expended to balance the equation. The following figures show percentages in the adult UK population of excess weight[6]:

- Women
  36% overweight
  12% obese

- Men
  45% overweight
  8% obese

Dietary advice on reducing caloric and fat intake combined with appropriate exercise advice is important for overweight CR patients in order to:

- Achieve an ideal BMI (of 20–25)
- Reduce cholesterol and triglyceride levels
- Normalize insulin and glucose levels
- Reduce blood pressure levels.

Cardiac rehabilitation groups are usually well motivated to lose weight and realistic target weights should be set with an average weight loss goal of 0.5–1.0 kg per week.

Losing weight is not easy as seen by the disappointing success rates in most of the population and the prevention of obesity, starting early in life, is of paramount importance in the general population. Dietary advice given to CR participants may have positive effects for the rest of the family, including a younger generation. Weight reduction needs support and encouragement from CR personnel, and any sustained weight loss should be noted and congratulated.

From the CHD viewpoint, *where* the fat is deposited is more interesting than obesity *per se*[7]. Fat deposited around the trunk, abdomen and internal organs, (apple shaped) influences the risk of CHD more than fat deposited peripherally about the hips and thighs (pear shaped). This central obesity (high waist to hip ratio) is associated with: an unfavourable lipid profile – high triglycerides/low HDL, reduced sensitivity to insulin, glucose intolerance, increase in plasma insulin and blood pressure – collectively known as syndrome X or Reaven's syndrome. This is treated by weight normalization and exercise.

Diet and diabetes mellitus

In both types of diabetes (insulin dependent and non-insulin dependent) there is an increased risk of CHD. The risk is associated with serum lipid levels, particularly the serum triglycerides, rather than related to blood glucose or glycaemic control[8]. Therefore, dietary measures should focus on modifying an abnormal lipid profile as well as blood glucose control.

Cardiovascular protective diet

A lipid-lowering diet is important for lowering plasma cholesterol but there are also protective dietary interventions such as anti-oxidants, soluble fibre and the synergistic interactions between dietary factors which need to be considered[9]. Therefore it is important to consider the diet as a whole and its positive cardio-protective action.

Total fat

Fat is a major component of many foods, providing energy, essential fatty acids and fat-soluble vitamins A, D and E. Fat is very calorie-dense providing approximately twice as much energy per gram as protein or carbohydrate. Therefore a high fat diet is high in energy and can predispose to a positive energy balance – overweight and obesity. Some fat is 'visible' and avoidable, i.e. in butter, margarines, oils, lard, shortenings, cream, cheese and meat; some fat is 'invisible', i.e. hidden in cakes, pastry, biscuits, crisps, processed meats and chocolate.

The present average intake of fat in the UK is too high, contributing 40% of the total energy intake. A reduction to 30–35% of total energy is recommended in the Committee on Medical Aspects of Food Policy (COMA) Report (1991), Dietary Reference Values for Food Energy and Nutrients for the United Kingdom[10].

Thrombogenic factors

More recently, Factor VII coagulant activity shows an acute increase after a fat-rich meal and a high Factor VII activity is sustained when the diet is habitually rich in fat. These increases can be reversed by a reduction in total fat intake. Factor VII coagulant activity has been shown to be a predictor of CHD risk[11].

Type of fat

Foods contain a mixture of different types of fat in varying quantities. No food has only one type of fat. The name used to describe a particular type of fat is determined because it contains mainly that type of fatty acids, e.g. olive oil is 'monounsaturated' because it contains 75% monounsaturated oleic acid but it also contains 14% saturated fatty acids and 11% polyunsaturated fatty acids.

Blood cholesterol levels are influenced by the type of fat in the diet[12]. Saturated fatty acids (SFA) raise plasma cholesterol while monounsaturated fatty acids (MUFA) and polyunsaturated fatty acids (PUFA) lower plasma cholesterol.

Saturated fatty acids

Saturated fatty acids are found principally in foods of animal origin: meat and meat products, dairy foods, biscuits, cakes, confectionery and spreading fats. Products which contain predominantly saturated fats are solid at room temperature. COMA (1991)[10] recommends that the saturated fatty acid composition of the diet should make up no more than 10% of the total energy, a reduction from the current 16% seen in the UK population.

Monounsaturated fatty acids (MUFA)

The main MUFA in the diet is oleic acid. It is the principal fatty acid found in olive oil and rapeseed oil but also a major component of fats in other vegetable oils, dairy products, meat, and is a major contributor to total fat intake. Other rich sources are nuts, oily fish and avocados. Within the limits of total fat intake, substitution of saturates by monounsaturates offers certain advantages and is consistent with the low incidence of CHD in Mediterranean populations who traditionally consume a diet low in saturates, but rich in olive oil.

Polyunsaturated fatty acids (PUFA)

There are two major types of PUFA in the diet, the omega-6 and omega-3 series: Ω-6 and Ω-3 series.

Omega-6 series

The predominant fatty acid is linoleic acid, an essential fatty acid; rich sources are found in corn oil, safflower oil, sunflower oil and soyabean oil and PUFA margarines. The present intake of Ω-6 PUFA has risen to 6% food energy and current recommendations suggest that the intake should not be increased as there is little evidence on the safety of diets containing more than 10% Ω-6 PUFA over a lifetime[13]. PUFA are susceptible to oxidation with adverse consequences but most seed oils are rich in vitamin E, a potent antioxidant. However, it is prudent for diets containing substantial amounts of PUFA to be adequately supplied with vitamin E.

Omega-3 series

The other essential fatty acid is linolenic acid found in green leaves, seeds and seed oil especially soya and rapeseed oil. Other types are found in oily fish and fish oils. The vital fatty acids in fish oil are eicosapentaenoic acid (EPA) and docosahexaenoic acid (DHA) (see Table 7.1).

Table 7.1   Quantity of PUFA(g) per 100 g oily fish

Oily fish	omega-3 PUFA (g/100 g)
Mackerel	2.2
Herring	1.7
Sardines	1.7
Pilchards	1.7
Trout (lake)	1.6
Salmon	1.4
Halibut	0.9
Trout (rainbow)	0.6
Tuna	0.5

A fishy tale

Fish oils reduce triglycerides and promote HDL cholesterol but the major effect of fish oils appears to be anti-thrombotic and anti-inflammatory. In the Diet and Re-infarction Trial (DART) (an intervention with men who had already had an MI), increasing the consumption of oily fish to two portions per week or consuming equivalent amount of fish oils resulted in a significant reduction in mortality from CHD and total mortality over the following two years[14]. Therefore the recommendation of oily fish twice per week or a fish oil supplement containing 800 mg of omega-3 daily (EPA + DHA) is important. Cod liver oil is as suitable as pure fish oils but does contain vitamins A and D, so should not be taken in excess.

Trans fatty acids (TFA)

Overall the average UK diet contains very little of this type of fat which contributes 2% of the total energy content of the UK diet. Current scientific evidence suggests trans fatty acids behave in a similar way to SFA but also have an undesirable effect on CHD mortality[15].

Trans fatty acids are formed during the hydrogenation process of liquid oils to hardened margarines and shortenings, and are found in products using these fats to make biscuits, pastries, pies, cakes, chips, processed dairy and meat products. There are also a small amount of trans fatty acids naturally from ruminant fat in beef, lamb and other meat products and dairy foods, butter and cheese.

Some concern regarding the trans fatty acid content of some PUFA margarines and low-fat spreads has recently come to the forefront and consequently some leading brands have been reformulated to reduce trans fatty acid content. It would be sensible to use all margarines and low fat spreads sparingly while remembering that most of the trans fatty acids in the diet come from commercially prepared, processed and baked products and emphasis should be given to ways of limiting these foods. In summary, the COMA Report on Dietary Reference Values (1991)[10] recommends the following balance of fats in the diet:

Saturated fatty acids	10%
Monounsaturated fatty acids	12%
Polyunsaturated fatty acids	6% (up to 10% maximum)
Trans fatty acids	2%.

Dietary cholesterol

Cholesterol is essential in the body, as:

- Part of the structure of cells;
- The basis of bile acids;
- The basis of some hormones, steroids and sex hormones, and vitamin D.

The influence of dietary cholesterol on plasma cholesterol varies between individuals but for most people dietary cholesterol has little or no effect on plasma cholesterol. Dietary cholesterol is associated with dietary saturates in the diet and dietary strategies to reduce saturates tend also to reduce dietary cholesterol[12]. Eggs and offal meats such as liver, sweetbreads and brain are the major sources of dietary cholesterol in the diet. The consumption of shell fish, prawns, lobster and mussels does not raise plasma cholesterol as cholesterol in shellfish is poorly absorbed[16].

Dietary carbohydrates

Complex (starch) and non-starch polysaccharides (NSP)

An increase in the consumption of complex carbohydrate (starchy) foods is necessary to facilitate the decrease of total and saturated fat in the diet. Decreasing total fat reduces the energy content of the diet which must be replaced with energy from complex carbohydrates or monounsaturated/polyunsaturated fats or both, or weight loss will occur – which may be unnecessary for some people.

A high complex carbohydrate diet consisting of cereals, bread, pasta, rice, potatoes needs to be increased from 45% to 50% of dietary energy (COMA 1994)[13]. Contrary to popular belief these foods are *not* fattening – it's the *added* fat that makes them fattening – and add bulk, nutrient value and satiety value to meals.

Non-starch polysaccharides (NSP) fibre

The general term used for fibre is non-starch polysaccharides (NSP) and the dietary reference value (DRV) for NSP is 18 g per day.

Insoluble fibre is found in wholegrain foods such as:

- Wholegrain bread
- Wheatgerm bread
- Granary bread
- Wholemeal flour
- Wholewheat pasta
- Brown rice
- Wholemeal noodles
- Wholewheat breakfast cereals.

Insoluble fibre

Insoluble fibre has been well documented for its effect on healthy digestion, helping to avoid constipation and diseases of the bowel. Enough fluid should be encouraged when taking a high fibre diet – 10 cups or 6 mugs per day.

Soluble fibre

Soluble fibre found in oats, pulses (beans and peas), fruit and vegetables lowers post-prandial insulin, glucose levels and LDL cholesterol[17]. Soluble fibre lowers LDL cholesterol by reducing the re-absorption of cholesterol-rich bile acids in the large bowel.

Non-milk extrinsic sugars (mainly sucrose)

Sugar does not have a causal link with CHD but can contribute to overweight and obesity by being calorie dense without any additional nutrients. Products containing high levels of sugar also tend to contain high levels of saturated fat. High intakes can have undesirable effects in dental health. Non-milk extrinsic sugars should not contribute to more than 10% of total energy[13].

The Mediterranean diet

Southern Mediterranean countries have less CHD than the UK despite similar plasma cholesterol levels, total fat intakes and a high incidence of smoking. The traditional 'Mediterranean' diet is rich in olive oil (high in monounsaturated fatty acids) and contains much more salads and fresh fruit and vegetables than are consumed in this country; it is seen as cardioprotective.

Anti-oxidant nutrients

Vitamins in fruit and vegetables are well known for their role in preventing classical defiency diseases but less for their role in the body's defences against oxygen free-radicals, which may initiate atherosclerosis[18].

The main anti-oxidant vitamins are vitamin A, vitamin C, vitamin E (the ACE vitamins) and essential trace elements, selenium, zinc, and manganese. Beta-carotene, a pro-vitamin (converted into vitamin A in the body) and other carotenoids, such as lutein and lycopene (present in large amounts in tomatoes), and flavonoids, present in red wine, tea and onions, also have anti-oxidant properties.

Take 5!

Fruit and vegetables are a rich source of vitamins, minerals and fibre. The World Health Organization (1990) has recommended a daily intake of 450 g (1 lb) fruit and vegetables per day to protect against CHD[19]. This would amount to five portions of fruit and vegetable daily plus potatoes and including about 25 g/1 oz of pulses, nuts and seeds (the latter especially for vegetarians). Smokers or recent smokers should be encouraged to eat more than five portions daily as smoking decreases plasma levels of vitamins C and E. However, high dose supplements of vitamins E and C are not yet to be recommended as evidence is not absolutely conclusive and there may be other substances in fruit and vegetables which are equally protective. There is a lot of interest in the role of anti-oxidant nutrients and much research is underway which will give further information.

Good sources of anti-oxidants

Vitamin E

Vitamin E has a protective effect on polyunsaturated fats both in food and in the body, preventing the oxidation of fats. Vitamin E requirement depends on the PUFA content of the diet but foods naturally high in PUFA are also naturally high in vitamin E. As dietary PUFA varies a lot, no dietary reference value is set for vitamin E but average daily intake is 5–10 mg per day. Supplements of vitamin E are much higher than this and do not appear to have adverse effects.

Good sources of vitamin E include: Vegetable oils, nuts (especially hazelnuts), oily fish (e.g. tuna), egg, wholewheat cereals, blackberries, avocado, spinach, asparagus, tomatoes, some margarines.

Vitamin C

Vitamin C is widely available in fruit and vegetables. It prevents scurvy, aids iron absorption and promotes wound healing. It also regenerates vitamin E. However, vitamin C is easily destroyed by cooking and will leach out into water, so fruit and vegetables should be eaten raw when possible to obtain plenty of vitamin C.

Dietary reference value (DRV): 40 mg daily.

Good sources of vitamin C include: Citrus fruits, citrus fruit juices, blackcurrants, strawberries, kiwi fruit, guava, paw paw, mango, melon, potatoes, peppers, cabbage, brussel sprouts, tomatoes, spinach.

Vitamin A and beta-carotene

Dietary vitamin A is measured as retinol-equivalent because, as well as the ready formed vitamin (retinol) in foods of animal origin, beta-carotene in plant foods is converted to retinol in the body:

$$6 \text{ mcg beta-carotene} \equiv 1 \text{ mcg retinol}$$

Vitamin A can be stored in the body and excessive amounts can be dangerous. It is important, therefore, that fish liver oils should be taken as per instructions on the label.

Dietary reference value:
600 mcg retinol/day for women
700 mcg retinol/day for men

Intakes should not exceed:
7500 mcg retinol/day for women
9000 mcg retinol/day for men

Beta carotene is the pigment that gives green, yellow and orange fruit and vegetables their colour.

Good sources of vitamin A as fat-soluble retinol include: Margarines, cheese, egg yolk, liver, fatty fish, fish liver oils.

Good sources of beta-carotene include: Carrots, lettuce, cabbage, spinach, spring greens, sweet potato, melon, mango, yellow and red fruits and vegetables.

Trace elements

Zinc: Found in many foods, but meat, unmilled cereals and pulses are particularly good sources.
Selenium: Content varies depending on the content in the soil for the crop and the animals, but good sources are: meat, fish, milk, eggs, wheat and bread.
Manganese: Found in whole cereals, pulses and leafy vegetables, and tea is a very rich source.

Alcohol

A number of studies have shown a relationship between alcohol consumption and low risk of CHD[20]. Alcohol intake is associated with higher levels of HDL cholesterol, lower levels of plasma fibrinogen and reduced platelet activity and hence a lower probability of thrombosis. However, alcohol can adversely affect cardiovascular disease as high blood pressure is related to habitual consumption of alcohol and rises with acute alcohol consumption.

The French paradox

There is a strong inverse association between national average wine consumption and national CHD mortality. Red wine, particularly, contains polyphenols which are a kind of flavonoid, not found in other alcoholic drinks, with anti-oxidant properties offering some protection against CHD, thus the 'French paradox'. Alcohol may provide many people with enjoyment but it is also linked to increased morbidity, mortality and social problems. The levels of consumption of alcohol recommended by the medical profession, as unlikely to cause harm to health, are 14 units weekly for women and 21 units weekly for men. One unit is defined as the equivalent of 8 g pure ethanol and found in one glass of wine, one measure of spirit or half a pint of beer. However, the balance of risk and benefit is against recommending the public to consume alcohol to lessen the risk of CHD.

Sodium

The average daily intake of salt (sodium chloride) in the UK is 10 g daily (2 teaspoons) and recommendations are to decrease this to 6 g by reducing or eliminating the amount of salt added to food in cooking or at the table. This discretionary salt amounts to one third of our daily intake. The other two-thirds is found in processed and manufactured foods. Particularly salty foods are processed meats, smoked foods, savoury snack foods, cheese, soups, convenience meals, some breakfast cereals and bread.

Potassium

To increase the potassium content of the diet and decrease the sodium–potassium ratio, a high intake of potassium is important and good sources are found in vegetables and fruit (especially bananas).

The cardioprotective diet

A range of foods can be recommended or discouraged for CR patients in general, and for those with specific dietary needs. See Appendix 5 for an outline of a cardioprotective diet and an outline of practical tips for preparing food. Common myths about eating according to a cardioprotective diet, e.g. raised costs, are also addressed in the Appendix. A list of useful publications on diet is also included following the references.

Myths

Cost

A healthy cardioprotective diet need not be more expensive than the average diet. A lot of healthier foods have a cost bonus added – e.g. lean meat, low fat cheeses, wholemeal bread, fresh fruit, etc. However, when balanced against the savings from replacing a lot of manufactured and processed foods with fresh basic foods, the total cost is comparable. The daily diet should be based around inexpensive starchy foods such as bread, rice, pasta, potatoes, flavoured with smaller and therefore cheaper portions of meat and fish. Seasonal fruit and vegetables are cheaper than exotic out-of-season varieties. Pulses make very cheap nutritious meals on their own or extending meat casseroles and stews.

Labelling

'Low fat' means that the product contains less than 5 g/fat per 100 g and the term 'reduced fat' means the product contains 25% less fat than the standard product.

Foods are labelled with the amount of fat in grams/100 g, the % fat, and, in some cases, the amount of SFA, MUFA and SFA.

Spreading fats

Butter and margarine contain the same amount of fat and food energy by law – of 80 g fat/100 g – and have the same number of calories; the type of fat differs. Low-fat-spreads contain about 40 g fat per 100 g and contain more water and so are less suitable for baking. Very-low-fat-spreads contain 20–25 g fat/100 g, and the most recent margarines contain 0–5% fat. Choosing a spreading fat is confusing for the consumer but one should be chosen that has low SFA content (less than 15 g of SFA per 100 g) so compare labels.

Garlic and onions

Garlic has been a panacea for centuries for a variety of ills. The principal bioactive ingredient is alliin, which on disruption of cloves is converted to allicin. Onions contain smaller amounts of alliin but also contain anti-oxidant flavonoids such as quercetin. Reported effects include inhibition of platelet aggregation, increase in fibrinolysis, reduction in plasma concentrations of fibrinogen, reduction of total and LDL-cholesterol and an increase in HDL-cholesterol. Evidence that garlic reduces cardiovascular risk factors is accumulating but is incomplete. In the meantime, it would seem reasonable to take plenty of garlic, if liked, either fresh or as a dried preparation.

Coffee

Evidence remains inconsistent: the Scandinavian practice of boiling coffee during its preparation appears to generate a hypercholesterolaemic fraction; however, coffee drinking as practised in the UK does not appear to affect CHD risk.

Tea

Tea drinkers have similar caffeine intakes to coffee drinkers. Recently, tea has been shown to contain a rich source of anti-oxidants (flavonoids) which may protect against CHD.

Milk

Skimmed milk should not be used for children under 2 years in the family; semi-skimmed milk is fine for 2–5-year olds and skimmed and semi-skimmed suitable for everyone else. Skimmed milks are lower in fat and energy and small children need more energy-dense foods. However, the calcium content of skimmed milk is comparable to that of semi-skimmed and full-fat milks.

Soft water

A weak inverse association between water hardness and cardiovascular disease mortality has been reported. Individual members of the public who soften water in their own homes may wish to take the precaution of drinking unsoftened water.

Motivation

People need to be enthusiastically motivated to change lifestyle behaviour, and changing the habits of a lifetime is never easy. The positive aspects of healthy eating need always to be emphasized and changes encouraged and supported by the CR team.

Summary of key points

- There is no such thing as good food or bad food and nothing is forbidden.
- It is the general everyday eating of a variety of foods which is important, and special occasions which prove the exception rather than the rule are perfectly normal.
- For long-term compliance, dietary changes should be made gradually, taking one step at a time at the individual pace of the patient and his or her family.
- New eating habits take a long time to learn and improvements in lipid profiles continue over periods of years as healthy eating becomes a way of life.
- Practical help with recipes, meal planning and food tasting are paramount for dietary success and can add a sense of fun and enjoyment to all concerned with cardiac rehabilitation.

References

1. National Academy of Sciences, Committee on Diet and Health (1989) *Diet and Health: Implications for Reducing Chronic Disease Risk*, Washington DC: National Academy Press.
2. Study Group of the European Atherosclerosis Society (1987) Strategies for the prevention of coronary heart disease: a policy statement of the European Atherosclerosis Society, *European Heart Journal*, **8**, 77–88.
3. Betteridge, D.J., Dodson, P.M., Durrington, P.N. *et al.* (1993) Management of hyperlipidaemia: guidelines of the British Hyperlipidaemia Association, *Postgraduate Medical Journal*, **69**, 359–69.
4. Castelli, W.P.(1986) The triglyceride issue: a view from Framingham, *American Heart Journal*, **112**, 432–37.

5. Intersalt Cooperative Research Group (1988) Intersalt: an international study of electrolyte excretion and blood pressure: results for 24-hour urinary sodium and potassium excretion, *British Medical Journal*, **297**, 319–28.
6. White, N., Nicolaas, G., Foster, K., Browne, F. and Carey, S. (1993) *Health Surveys for England 1991: A survey carried out by the Social Survey Division of the OPCS on behalf of the Department of Health*, London: HMSO.
7. Ducimetière, P., Richard, J. and Cambien, F. (1986) The pattern of distribution of subcutaneous fat distribution in middle-aged men and the risk of coronary heart disease: the Paris prospective study, *International Journal of Obesity*, **10**, 229–40.
8. West, K.M., Ahuja, M.M. *et al.* (1983) The role of circulating glucose and triglyceride concentrations and their interactions with other risk factors as determinants of arterial disease in nine diabetic population samples from the WHO multinational study, *Diabetes Care*, **6**, 361–9.
9. Ulbricht, T.L.V. and Southgate, D.A.T. (1991) Coronary heart disease: seven dietary factors, *Lancet*, **338**, 985–92.
10. Department of Health, Committee on Medical Aspects of Food Policy (1991) *Dietary Reference Values for Food Energy and Nutrients for the United Kingdom: Report of the Panel on Dietary Reference Values. Report on Health and Social Subjects No 41*, London: HMSO.
11. Meade, T.W., Mellows, S., Brozovic, M. *et al.* (1986) Haemostatic function and ischaemic heart disease: principle results of the Northwick Park Heart Study, *Lancet*, **2**, 533–7.
12. Hegsted, D.M., Ausman, L., Johnson, J.A. *et al.* (1993) Dietary fat and serum lipids: an evaluation of the experimental data, *American Journal of Clinical Nutrition*, **57**, 875–83.
13. Department of Health, Committee on Medical Aspects of Food Policy (1994) *Nutritional Aspects of Cardiovascular Disease*, London: HMSO.
14. Burr, M.L., Fehily, A.M., Giulbert, J.F. *et al.* (1989) Effects of changes in fat, fish and fibre intakes on death and myocardial infarction: Diet and re-infarction trial (DART), *Lancet*, **2**, 757–61.
15. Ascherio, A., Hennekens, C.H., Buring, J.E., Master, C., Stampfer, M.J. and Willett, W.C. (1994) Trans-fatty acids intake and risk of myocardial infarction, *Circulation*, **89**, 94–101.
16. Connor, W.E. and Lin, D.S. (1982) The effect of shellfish in the diet upon the plasma lipid level in humans, *Metabolism*, **31**, 1046–51.
17. Ripsin, C.M., Keenan, J.M., Jacobs, D.R., Elmer, P.J., Welch, R.R. *et al.* (1992) Oat products and lipid lowering: a meta analysis, *Journal of the American Medical Association*, **267**, 3317–25.
18. Steinberg, D. (1993) Antioxidant vitamins and coronary heart disease, *New England Journal of Medicine*, **328**, 1487–89.
19. World Health Organization. (1990) *Diet, Nutrition and the Prevention of Chronic Diseases: Report of a WHO Study Group*, Geneva: Technical report series 797, WHO.

20. Marmot, M.G. (1984) Alcohol and coronary heart disease, *International Journal of Epidemiology*, **13**, 160–7.

Suggestions for further reading

Ashwell, M. (ed.) (1994) *Diet and Heart Disease*, London: British Nutrition Foundation.

Ball, M. and Mann, J. (1988) *Lipids for Heart Disease: A Practical Approach*, London: The Family Heart Association.

Durrington, P.N. (1989) *Hyperlipidaemia – Diagnosis and Management*, Bristol: John Wright.

Longstaff, R. and Mann, J. (1986) *The Healthy Heart Diet Book*, London: Optima Positive Health Guides.

National Dairy Council Nutrition Service (1992) *Coronary Heart Disease 1 and II – Fact File 7 and 8*.

Sanders, T. (1994) *Dietary Fats: A Nutrition Briefing Paper*, London: Health Education Authority.

Recipe books

Lindsay, A. (1994) *The Light Hearted Cook Book*, London: British Heart Foundation.

Lynas, J. (1994) *The Heart of Delicious Cooking*, Surrey: Pulse Medical Publishing Ltd.

Marshall, J. and Heughan, A. (1992) *Eat For Life Diet*, London: Vermilion.

Saynor, R. and Ryan, F. (1990) *The Eskimo Diet Cookbook*, London: Ebury Press.

Symes, D. and Zakary, A. (1991) *Low-Fat Diet Book*, London: The Family Heart Association.

Chapter 8

Funding Issues in Cardiac Rehabilitation

Summary

This chapter is concerned with funding issues and although written principally for cardiac rehabilitation (CR) programme managers in both community and hospital settings in the NHS, it may also be useful reference material for those providing CR in the independent sector and those collaborating organizations, such as the British Heart Foundation (BHF) and the Coronary Prevention Group (CPG). The aim is to help programme managers construct the financial element of their service proposals – using valid clinical arguments to support the need for services and demonstrating the cost effectiveness of provision to service purchasers and funding agencies.

A systematic approach is essential in the competitive, but financially constrained, world of health care in the UK, where NHS purchasing authorities determine priorities of need in local populations and award contracts conditionally to successful 'bidders' for all manner of different services. As experience has shown that purchasers may wish, in some instances, to give only partial financial support to CR proposals, service providers need to identify other sources of finance and to develop funding options that are not solely dependent on the NHS purchasing authority.

Programme managers need information to enable them to put forward their proposals as strongly as possible. This includes:

- Understanding the purchaser/provider relationship in funding services;
- Justifying the investment;
- Types of contract;
- Costing the service and building a budget;

- Sources of funding;
- Charitable status.

The purchaser/provider relationship

The National Health Service and Community Care Act 1990 introduced far-reaching changes in the management of the NHS. A split was made between NHS purchasers of care – the District Health Authority (DHA) Health Commissions, Family Health Service Authorities (FHSA) and GP fundholders – on the one hand, and the NHS providers of health care on the other. NHS providers are NHS Trusts, i.e. hospitals and community health units, and directly managed units (DMUs), i.e. hospitals and community units which are not yet trusts and are therefore accountable to the DHA.

The 'internal market' was created in which providers would compete to win purchaser contracts for particular services. Other providers outside the NHS, such as private or independent hospitals and nursing homes, could also compete for service contracts, thus widening the scope of competition beyond the 'internal market'.

Purchaser responsibilities

The DHA, as a purchasing authority, has a primary duty to buy health services from providers on behalf of the population it serves, based on prevailing needs and available resources. Inevitably, the purchaser must determine priorities and discussions with prospective providers will play a key role in decision-making.

Specific functions of the purchasing authority include:

- Consulting the population served on their needs and satisfaction with service;
- Identifying the health needs of the population served;
- Planning patterns of provision and purchasing strategy in the longer term;
- Collaborating with local providers (hospitals, nursing and residential homes, statutory providers such as social services, and voluntary organizations) to plan services;
- Determining the range and level of services to be purchased annually;
- Awarding contracts to providers with specifications covering volume, quality standards and price.

Provider responsibilities

NHS health services are commonly referred to as hospital or community or primary care (GP) services. NHS providers, whether DMUs or trusts differ in the constellation of services they provide. A common division is between acute general hospital services and community health services – the latter often including mental health, learning disability, district nursing and health visiting. CR services may be located in either. It often depends on who got things going in the first place!

Providers have particular responsibilities. These are:

- Managing the delivery of the services they are under contract to provide within agreed quality standards, volume and price;
- Ensuring compliance with statutory orders and financial instructions;
- Securing sufficient income to cover the cost of service provision;
- Contributing to the development of local health plans and purchasing strategies with purchasers;
- Collaborating with purchasers and other providers to achieve co-ordinated provision of services for individual patients (packages of care);
- Determining user-satisfaction with services provided.

Justifying the investment

Traditionally there has been a tendency for CR services to be established by pioneers (doctors, nurses and therapists) who have sought in due time to persuade management in the NHS to fund the service on a permanent basis. Success in developing and maintaining CR services has been varied. Some services are fully funded by purchasers, some partially funded and some not funded at all. There continues to be controversy about the priority that purchasers should give to developing CR services and what they should encompass if they are to be provided.

Those responsible for managing CR services have the necessary task of persuading purchasers to fund these programmes. They need to show purchasers the real benefits (outcomes) of CR to patients and close carers alike, and to link the benefits (service effectiveness) to cost-effectiveness and efficiency (value for money). Illustrating what should go into a programme, e.g. that secondary and tertiary prevention strategies might include the patient's family as well as the patient, will not of itself justify service provision from the purchaser's viewpoint. Programme managers need to support their proposals with arguments that answer questions that the purchasers use to help them determine priorities.

Measures of the effectiveness of CR programmes

Purchasers may want to have evidence, preferably research based, which will show health benefits to patients and value for money.

For example:

- Measurable health gains from CR programmes:
  - □ Increased physical fitness and endurance as shown by an increase in functional capacity[1];

- □ Increased anginal thresholds – can patients perform more exercise with less angina, and learn to manage their anginal pain?[2]
- □ Psychological gains – increased well-being, decreased depression and anxiety[3];
- □ Socioeconomic gains, for example, are patients returning to work sooner?[4]
- □ Health promotion – can the ripple effect of health promotion be demonstrated in the families of cardiac patients by the evidence of change in their lifestyles? Are patients and their families smoking less, taking more exercise, eating a healthier diet than before? (This could have an effect on other services, e.g. by reducing incidence of cancer and osteoporosis);
- □ Risk factor intervention – effectiveness and timeliness is important for optimizing recovery of the patient, e.g. accurate cholesterol testing and appropriate advice, applied at the right time[4,5];
- □ Reduced morbidity and mortality[6].
- ■ Cost effectiveness:
  - □ Fewer hospital re-admissions;
  - □ Reduced medications;
  - □ Higher return to work rates.
- ■ Efficiency:
  - □ Cost per patient as compared to other intervention.

Types of contract

NHS contracts are based currently on one of these types:

- ■ Block contracts
- ■ Cost and volume contracts
- ■ Cost per case contracts.

Block contracts are the simplest forms of contracting and are based on a fixed sum of money being agreed for an indicative volume of service, for an agreed period. If the contract is agreed to cover a period of one year then equal twelfths will be paid on a monthly basis no matter how the workload fluctuates on a month by month basis, or in total over the full year of the contract.

Cost and volume contracts cover a specified volume of service for a fixed sum of money. With this type of contract an agreed sum of money is typically being paid for a specified level of quality with differing prices being paid for variations in the actual level of service provided or below the agreed target. Cost per case contracts cover agreements where each unit of activity leads to an agreed level of payment.

Costing service provision and building a budget

While setting out the benefits of a CR programme is a critical part of negotiating for funds, the programme manager will also need to be clear about the level of service needed and prepare a detailed analysis of the cost of provision. The demand for the service should be supported by data supplied from sources such as local public health departments, the NHS Management Executive, other CR services, and sources such as the Coronary Prevention Group and the British Heart Foundation. Purchasers, too, will be taking into account this kind of data in deciding whether to purchase the service.

Within the NHS, the price of services is based on the principle that cost equals price. Cardiac rehabilitation services would not be expected to make a profit. During 1993 the Department of Health (DoH) introduced a standard approach to costing services within the NHS with the intention of achieving consistency in provider analysis of their costs, which would provide comparability of costs among providers on an equitable basis.

The three main areas of cost are:

- Fixed costs: those which are not affected by changes in any one year, e.g. capital depreciation, capital charges, rent or rates;
- Semi-fixed costs: those which vary when specified increases or decreases in levels of activity are reached. For example, staffing levels remain unchanged when there is an increase or decrease in the number of patients being treated until the specified level has been reached;
- Variable costs: those which vary with each individual activity, e.g. the number of electrodes used or the number of cholesterol tests performed in one year.

Various factors affecting cost need to be considered:

- Service demand: Can referral rates be projected? How many CR users annually?
- Level of service: Does the programme consist of exercise alone or is stress management and/or health education included as part of the package?
- Frequency of service: How many times per week do patients attend, and for how many weeks?
- Staffing levels: How many members are there in the CR team? Does the service fluctuate during holiday periods or sickness?
- Equipment: What apparatus is used? What is its shelf-life? Who is responsible for maintenance of a defibrillator, for example? Depreciation costs?
- Administration costs: Is secretarial support necessary? Are there photocopying facilities or is a telephone account associated with the programme?
- Accommodation and leases: Is this provided free of charge or is there a rental charged?

The analysis of these factors will enable the CR manager to produce a service programme specification which quantifies the staff and non-staff resources that will be required to deliver the programme. The cost per patient can be calculated by dividing the total cost of the programme by the estimated number of patients referred to and participating in the programme annually.

Building a CR programme budget

A budget is an agreed statement of the probable allocation and use of funds over a year. Budgets will usually take into account the cost analysis headings of direct, indirect and overheads as well as the fixed, semi-fixed and variable costs already mentioned.

Direct costs are controlled directly by the budget holder. Indirect costs and overheads are a shared element of any organization's costs, such as the general management team, the power supply or the cost of a building. Budget holders are accountable for those costs which they control.

Any budget for a department will be broken down to recognize this analysis within the function of the department concerned. It will also identify the planned level of funding and expenditure for each element. An example of this could be the type of staff employed or the supplies costs for consumables used, or the cost of stationery generated purely by the CR department. Included in the overall cost of the service is the CR programme's share of the costs of the general management team, use of hospital and corridor space, for example, and even the hospital grounds in some instances.

The person managing the budget will require details forecasting expenditure of the period in question and also knowledge of the true costs at the present time. This means that where contracts are concerned, specific levels of income have been correctly forecast, and that the activity levels have been met. If the forecast level of activity is not met, the income will vary in all but the simplest form of block contract.

Once service activity levels and quality standards have been specified the programme manager needs to build up the different cost components of the budget.

Essentially there are:

- Staff costs;
- Consumables and equipment costs;
- Costs of services including rents and recharges between departments.

Salary and salary-related costs are likely to be a major part of the total CR budget. Depending on the circumstances, the following is a list of what needs to be considered[7]:

- Basic salary costs (determined by establishment);

- Clinical grade of each post;
- Pay point of individuals; incremental dates;
- (London weighting);
- Annual cost-of-living increase.

Allowances will also have to be made for the following:

- Special duty payments (eg. unsocial hours);
- Overtime;
- Annual leave;
- Sickness;
- Maternity leave;
- Acting up;
- Training.

Staff related costs:

- National Insurance employer's contribution;
- Superannuation: employer's contribution;
- Leased car: employer's costs;
- Mileage allowances;
- Performance-related pay;
- Crèche.

Information on the actual costs applicable can be obtained from the finance department of the provider.
Non-staff costs cover:

- Consumables
  drugs
  dressings
  catering provision
  uniforms
  stationery, including patient leaflets/handouts and photocopying
  CSSD (Central Sterile Supplies Dept)
  disposable linen
- Equipment
  medical and surgical supplies
  appliances
  crockery and cutlery
- Services
  laundry
  domestics
  cleaning

telephone/communications
maintenance contracts.

Sources of funding and investment

Some of the more common means of generating income include services provided to an individual patient from outside any residential areas covered by contracts or to GP fundholders, from supporting work to private hospitals, or separately agreed private patients.

Alternative sources of funding may therefore include:

- Extra contractual referrals (ECRs) and tertiary referrals;
- GP fundholders;
- Private patients;
- Fund-raising activities;
- Patient donations;
- Bids for health gains;
- Sponsorship;
- Research.

Extra contractual referrals, tertiary referrals and GP fundholders

Patients who do not reside in the health district of their nearest CR programme or the programme of their own or their doctor's choosing may be considered to be an extra contractual referral (ECR). There are three classifications of ECR – emergency, elective and tertiary referral. In the instance of emergency or tertiary referrals treatment must be consented to by the appropriate authority, who have the right to be notified of the details and costs of the treatment **before treatment commences**. An account, with supporting information, must be submitted to the paying authority within an agreed time span, e.g. 6 weeks. When a patient is referred by a hospital consultant for specialist care at a specialist centre – such as a cardiac centre or a CR unit – the referral is classed as 'tertiary'. For elective care, consent must be obtained by the organization providing the treatment, before treatment is provided.

In summary, it is the health authority where the patient resides which is usually responsible for paying for the cost of treatment (unless the patient's doctor is a fundholder) but this needs to be 'authorized' or agreed so that money changes hands prior to the commencement of treatment. When a patient is referred for rehabilitation by a hospital consultant, this is deemed to be a 'tertiary referral'. Referrals carrying this status imply that payment to the provider by the patient's health authority is mandatory. The hospital consultant making the referral needs to complete a standard form PU1 to authorize treatment, prior to the patient being invited to attend the programme. This form is sent to the paying health authority, which re-imburses the provider unit the cost of the treatment episode.

GP fundholders

Some general practitioners contract directly with hospital or community providers for defined services. In these circumstances the fundholders will receive the appropriate share of the health authority's allocation for the defined services. They agree specific contracts for the provision of services. Such agreements are currently quite explicit regarding the volume and nature of the service provided and tend to be cost per case agreements.

If a GP fundholder refers a patient to a CR programme , the GP fundholder is responsible for payment to the provider. In addition, GP fundholders may wish to purchase the CR service for several patients and take out a block contract with the provider unit. In some instances they may prefer to purchase diagnostic exercise tests from CR units rather than using hospital ECG departments – particularly if the latter has a longer waiting list. It would seem reasonable to charge the same rate as the hospital for this service.

Private patients

It is possible to levy individual charges on private patients within the provider organization, as a part of a special private patient service. Most purchasers will support such services being offered provided that the private patients do not receive preferential treatment which would disadvantage non-fee-paying patients.

Private patients' insurance policies are another potential source of income. BUPA, PPP and other schemes offer their clients re-imbursement for exercise ECG tests and sometimes for rehabilitation courses. It is good practice not to enforce payment on private patients but encourage them to claim from their policies where possible. What is a reasonable fee to levy on such patients? It is probably best to decide upon a sum that is less than the market price per capita but greater than the true cost per case. Private patients attending CR alongside NHS patients do not receive superior treatment, particularly in a class format. It is unfair therefore in these circumstances to charge exorbitant fees.

Fund-raising activities

Most CR programmes become involved in raising funds at some stage. It can be hugely time-consuming unless entirely patient-led, but has many rewards that include raising the profile of CR as a whole and fostering camaraderie between patients and the CR staff members. All fund-raising efforts should pass the following test:

The financial gain achieved must exceed the effort expended.

There are several ways to raise public awareness and to promote CR programmes. Designing a 'logo' to be used on a multitude of items for sale or distributed freely could be a starting point. This gives the CR scheme an identity. Following on from logos comes designing T-shirts, sweatshirts and other items, such as writing paper, sponsor forms, biros and advertisements which sport the logo and elevate the service's profile. Starter funds must be available to resource this type of venture. Donations from grateful patients, for example, can be placed in a hospital trust fund (earning interest), and be used to pump-prime fund-raising initiatives.

Patients and their families and friends may be willing to take part in a variety of events such as fun-runs, for which they can seek sponsorship. Healthy types of events are particularly attractive as they reinforce the health promotion message. Larger scale events, ranging from concerts, barn dances, car boot sales or auctions, and staged at different times during the year are also excellent money-spinners. These activities require a willing band of volunteers to mastermind and organize them. Although there are many excellent ways of raising money it is unwise to make the CR staff responsible for co-ordinating these events. The Lions or Rotary Clubs are often willing to help run local projects and share the fund-raising burden with ex-patients, particularly when the effort is directed towards an explicit and definable target such as buying a certain piece of equipment for the CR unit.

Patient donations

Many patients will show their gratitude to the CR team by donating a small or sometimes large sum of money, upon completion of the rehabilitation course. These donations, if placed in a hospital trust fund, will accrue interest which can be used to enhance any aspect of the CR programme. If the CR unit is fortunate to have gained charitable status, donations can be placed in special charity accounts. It must be stressed that the merit of these donations lies substantially in their voluntary nature. Any efforts to 'encourage' such activities from most patients is both completely inappropriate and likely to be less than satisfactory.

Bids for health gains/Pump-priming

Sometimes development bids can be a source of income, either from Health Commissions or from the larger charitable organizations. Specific projects which identify definite outcomes are more likely to receive donations from this source. For example the British Heart Foundation has, since 1989, donated £25 000 to pump-prime selected new CR programmes over their first two-year periods.

Sponsorship

As a means of covering service costs, sponsorship is sought in a number of different ways. This may be done by advertising on department stationery to offset the cost of its production, by fund-raising for equipment, or using drug company sponsorship to help fund research.

Some units manage to acquire sponsorship from industry to help keep their financial state robust. Drug companies may also wish to become involved with the programme – or a particular aspect of what is done which relates directly to their work. The food industry may wish to align itself with healthy messages about nutrition, or sporting companies might support the exercise component of CR. Although sponsorship is widely used as a way of attracting additional income, and meeting the operating costs of services provided, careful thought needs to be given to moral or ethical considerations such as: 'Does the sponsorship promote unhealthy practices, e.g. smoking? Does it provide an unfair competitive edge in a market where there is strong competition? Moreover, does it force the CR unit to promote a particular product for an indefinite length of time? Purchasers and providers are much more aware of these issues today than in the past and are careful to ensure that bias and undue influence do not arise from sponsorships.

Research

Research is an integral part of the future development of CR. As such, it should not be primarily considered in terms of it's fund-raising potential. It can be possible, however, to boost funding temporarily by obtaining a grant towards a specific research project. Research funding can only be expected to cover the extra costs of completing the project and an appropriate level of overhead support. CR programmes may also link with other, e.g. university, departments where students wish to conduct applied research, rather than apply directly to grant-awarding bodies for funds.

Charitable status

Many organizations apply each year to the Charity Commissioners to become a registered charity, and consequently receive 'charitable status'. As an established programme expands it may be worth considering this concept, as a means of obtaining additional financial advantages, e.g. VAT exemptions or tax benefits. The decision to become a registered charity should not be taken lightly as often more, rather than less, work is created. Issues surrounding the employment of staff by a charity can of themselves produce many problems.

At least two CR units in the UK are established registered charities. Further information on this topic may be obtained by contacting either of the people detailed below:

Mr Russell Tipson
c/o Action Heart
117 Wellington Road
Dudley
West Midlands DY1 1UB

Tel: 01384 230222

Mrs Sally Turner
c/o Rehab
Alton Health Centre
Anstey Road
Alton, Hants GU34 2QX

Tel: 01420 544794

Summary of key points

- There are frequent changes in government policy which CR managers and budget holders need to take into full account when determining local provision for cardiac rehabilitation.
- It is important that patients receive effective treatment which is delivered in a cost-efficient manner.
- Managers should resist compromising the standards of treatment simply in the interests of reducing costs.
- The challenge for the CR team in using the guidelines in this chapter will be to respond creatively to rising demands for services, with proposals which demonstrate effective treatment and efficient financial management.

References

1. Bethell, H. and Mullee, M. (1990) A controlled trial of community-based coronary rehabilitation, *British Heart Journal*, **64**, 370–5.
2. Todd, I. and Ballantyne, D. (1990) Antianginal efficacy of exercise training: a comparison with beta blockade, *British Heart Journal*, **64**, 14–19.
3. Taylor, C., Houston-Miller, N., Ahn, D.K. *et al.* (1986) Effects of exercise programs on psychosocial improvement in uncomplicated postmyocardial infarction patients, *Journal of Psychosomatic Research*, **30**, 581–630.
4. Houston-Miller, N., Barr Taylor, C., Davidson, D., *et al.* (1991) The efficacy of risk factor intervention and psychosocial aspects of cardiac rehabilitation. In: *Guidelines for Cardiac Rehabilitation Programs*, American Association of Cardiovascular and Pulmonary Rehabilitation, pp. 89–103.
5. Department of Health (1993) Coronary Heart Disease and Stroke – key area handbook, January 1993, Chapter 4, para 20, p. 38.
6. O'Connor, G., Buring, J., Yusuf, S. *et al.* (1989) An overview of randomised trials of rehabilitation with exercise after myocardial infarction, *Circulation*, **80**, 234–44.
7. *Using Information in Managing the Nursing Resource* (1991) Financial management 5 regional consortium, North West Thames RHA in conjunction with Greenhalgh & Company Ltd, Publishers, London.

Phases of Cardiac Rehabilitation

Phase One: In-patient

Entry criteria	Exclude	Content	Time scale	Resources	Staffing	Location
■ Acute myocardial infarction (AMI); ■ Coronary artery bypass surgery; ■ Percutaneous transluminal coronary angioplasty; ■ Angina; ■ Other, e.g. heart failure, valve surgery, transplant surgery according to local policies.	No need to exclude anyone from this phase; No age limit.	Coronary care unit (CCU)/ward visits – Include partner/family; Reassurance; Information/education; Mobilization; Discharge planning; **Assessment includes:** ■ Family/personal history ■ Risk factor assessment ■ Prognostic evaluation ■ Risk stratification* ■ Psychosocial status ■ Socio-economic status ■ Vocational/leisure activities.	5–7 days (average) post-AMI; Length of hospital stay will vary according to diagnosis and treatment; **Exit criteria:** discharge from hospital.	Written and verbal information; Individual plan for care and lifestyle change; Discharge plan.	CCU staff; Medical staff; Ward staff; Specialized CR staff; Occupational therapist; Social worker.	Hospital.

* Not all of the information required for this may be available at this stage.

Phase Two: Immediate post-discharge

Entry criteria	Exclude	Content	Time scale	Resources	Staffing	Location
As before; Direct GP referrals; Self-referrals.	As before; May need to exclude those with psychiatric disorders from groups, if disruptive in a group setting.	Post-discharge follow-up; Surveillance: may identify deterioration or non-compliance with treatment; Further assessment/ investigation; Education	4–6 weeks; **Exit criteria:** flexible according to individual progress.	Telephone; Facilities for counselling/group sessions; Audio-visual aids; Written material	Multi-disciplinary CR team; Primary healthcare team.	Hospital site; Home; Community facilities.

Phase Three: Intermediate outpatient

Entry criteria	Exclude	Content	Time scale	Resources	Staffing	Location
Depends on content of programme. Those, unable to participate at all in an exercise programme should be included in other appropriate components depending on their individual needs.	Those who are unstable and require further investigation; Those with psychiatric conditions who may endanger themselves or others in an exercise situation.	Individual exercise prescription, based on: ■ clinical status; ■ risk stratification; ■ assessment of previous physical activity and future needs; Supervised exercise sessions; Home exercise programmes; Education, if not available previously; Vocational assessment.	6–12 weeks according to local policy and individual progress; **Exit criteria:** patient objectives may include: ■ understanding the benefits of exercise; ■ safe use of equipment if used; ■ knowledge of personal limits; ■ ability to monitor safe levels of exercise; ■ able to exercise symptom-free.	Safe exercise facilities; Adequate resuscitation resources.	Safe ratio of staff to patients depending on risk levels in the group; Staff who have necessary resuscitation skills; Staff who possess knowledge of exercise prescription;	Hospital or community setting.

Phase Four: Long-term maintenance

Entry criteria	Exclude	Content	Time scale	Resources	Staffing	Location
Those who have completed a supervised exercise programme; Those who could not complete an exercise programme.	Not applicable.	Maintenance of exercise and other lifestyle changes; Monitoring for risk factor change and secondary prevention; Monitoring of adherence to therapy; Vocational support.	Life-long commitment; **Exit criteria:** need to rejoin earlier phases.	Ongoing facilities for exercise; Cardiac support group.	CR team – liaison role; Primary healthcare team; Other community based staff, i.e. health promotion, sports centre, etc.	Community facilities; Home.

Audit Criteria

Minimum data set

- Total number of referrals;
- Diagnosis (AMI, CABG, PTCA, angina, heart failure, etc.);
- Referral source;
- Age;
- Gender;
- Ethnic origin;
- Number of re-admissions and reason;
- Number of deaths.

Risk stratification

- Percentage of patients undergoing post-myocardial infarction exercise testing;
- Percentage of patients undergoing post-myocardial infarction perfusion imaging;
- Percentage of patients receiving left ventricular function assessment by echocardiography or radionuclide ventriculogaphy.

Further diagnostic testing and intervention

- Percentage of patients receiving diagnostic coronary arteriography;
- Percentage of patients receiving CABG;
- Percentage of patients receiving PTCA;
- Interventions performed per patient hours during the programme for:
  angina
  dysrhythmia
  heart failure
  cardiac arrest.

Patients still experiencing angina at the end of the programme should be recorded. The percentage of such patients receiving diagnostic coronary arteriography should also be recorded.

Counselling or exercise sessions

- Percentage of eligible patients attending sessions;
- Percentage of eligible patients who drop out;
- Percentage of eligible female patients attending;
- Percentage of eligible patients of ethnic origin other than UK attending;
- Mean increment in fitness or effort tolerance by functional testing achieved in the programme;
- Frequency of minor and major cardiac complications during patient-hours of exercise;
- Frequency of minor and major orthopaedic complications per patient-hours of exercise.

Therapeutics and risk factor modification

- Percentage of patients taking aspirin;
- Percentage of patients taking beta-blockade;
- Percentage of patients taking ACE inhibitors;
- Percentage of patients taking or needing to use sublingual nitrate therapy;
- Number and percentage of patients attending (e.g. at follow-up exercise test) with systolic blood pressure > 160 mmHg or diastolic blood pressure > 90 mmHg at rest;
- Percentage of patients losing weight in the programme;
- Percentage of patients by pre-specified protocol (e.g. < age 75) who have had plasma lipids including HDL cholesterol measured;
- Percentage of patients receiving follow-up lipid assessment;
- Percentage of patients showing a decrease in plasma LDL or increase in plasma HDL cholesterol during the programme and follow-up;
- Percentage of patients showing decrease in plasma triglyceride during follow-up;
- Frequency of lipid assessment in relatives (particularly where high levels appear to be the only risk factor for coronary artery disease);
- Percentage of patients receiving lipid-lowering medication;
- Percentage of patients recording smoking cessation in short- and long term; (Ideally the self-reported figure should be compared with an objective measure such as exhaled CO measurement);
- Percentage of patients with psychosocial dysfunction (anxiety, depression, other) and percentage referred for further specialized counselling;
- Percentage of patients experiencing return to work problems.

Appendix 3

General Warm-up Suitable for a CR Class

Movement	Purpose	Coaching points
March on the spot 20 × alternate R & L legs.	To gradually increase metabolic demand. Also to mobilize hip and knee joints.	Remind about good posture. Arms should be relaxed and swinging naturally in cadence with marching.
Take feet about hip width apart and relax the knees slightly. Remind about straight backs & importance of holding abdomen in.		
Raise & lower shoulders (as in a shrug) × 8.	To mobilize the shoulder joints.	Keep the head central and still. Control the movement during raising *and* lowering.
Put the right hand on the R shoulder and circle the shoulder backwards × 4 and forwards × 4. Repeat with L shoulder.	To mobilize the shoulder joints.	Encourage isolation of the joint being mobilized, i.e. restrict movement in the rest of the body as much as possible so that the focus is on the shoulder action.
Tilt head R × 4 and than L × 4 (as if trying to place the ear on top of the shoulder). Then look R × 4 and L × 4 (as if looking behind).	To mobilize the cervical joints of the spine.	Encourage shoulders to be down and relaxed – discourage tendency to hunch shoulders in effort to perform the movement 'better'.
March again, alternate legs × 20.	Continue to increase metabolic demand.	Swing the arms a bit more this time.
Take feet apart again		
Bend sideways: R × 4, L × 4.	To mobilize thoracic and lumbar sections of spine.	Try not to lean forward or back. Support weight as you bend to right by placing R hand on side of R thigh. Do not 'bounce' in effort to get further over.
Turn trunk to look behind then face front again. Repeat R × 4, L × 4.	To mobilize thoracic and lumbar sections of spine.	Keep the knees slightly relaxed and hips facing forward.

Movement	Purpose	Coaching points
Raise alternate knees and touch opposite hand to knee. Repeat R & L × 20.	Continue to increase metabolic demand.	Back should be straight, discourage tendency to bend forward rather than raise the knee.
Stand, feet together. Point R foot forward × 4. Repeat L. Repeat action but now with heel to floor rather than toe, R & L × 4.	To mobilize ankle joint.	

Before stretches do some more 'pulse raising' movements

4 Steps to right closing feet between each step. Return to left. Repeat R & L several times. Walk forward for 4 steps clapping hands on last step. Walk backwards for 4 with clap. Repeat several times. Finish with more marching on spot.		N.B. If coordination is very poor stick to variations of marching on spot and knee raising

---

Stretches

Calf Stretch

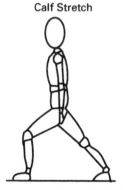

Keep weight central; make sure heel of back foot is down and toe is pointing forwards.

Back of thigh

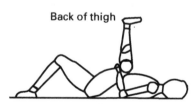

Back and hips must remain on the floor. Straighten leg gradually until stretch is felt at back of thigh.

Front of thigh

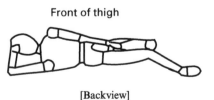

[Backview]

Bring foot in toward bottom until stretch is felt at front of thigh. Do not arch back. Keep thighs together

Upper chest

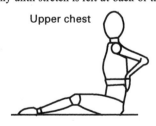

Retain good posture; don't allow the chin to poke forward.

Stretches

Back of arm

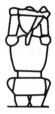

[Backview]

Do not arch back or allow chin to poke forward.
Those with poor shoulder mobility may have to
omit this stretch.

Hold each stretch for about 8–10 seconds.

Figures: courtesy of **Health Education Authority**.

Circuit Training Suitable for Inclusion in a CR Programme

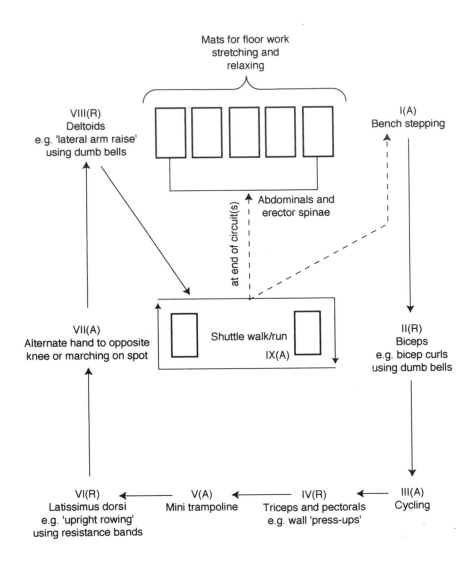

Circuit design considerations:

(1) Aerobic stations [A] and active recovery stations [R] should alternate.
(2) Based on individual prescription, aerobic activity should progress mainly through increased duration (30 s to 3 min at any one station is recommended). Progression may also be achieved through increased intensity by increasing stepping height [station I], pedal resistance [II], range of movement [V & VII] and speed [IX].
(3) Since the emphasis is on improving cardiovascular endurance (for which duration is the key factor) the duration of active recovery exercises (recommended 30 s) will not alter. Progression may, however, be achieved by increasing resistance, e.g. the use of stronger bands and/or heavier dumb bells.
(4) In group situations, the time spent at each 'aerobic' station will vary between individuals. Consequently, stations must be able to accommodate more than one participant at a time. If equipment is limited, e.g. trampolines or bicycles, other exercises which involve large muscle groups in rhythmic dynamic activity should be substituted.
(5) Upright aerobic work alternating with exercises performed in the supine position should be avoided. Hence abdominal and erector spinae exercises are performed in a group after the 9-station circuit(s) has/have been completed. A short period of low intensity activity, e.g. marking time on the spot, is recommended before commencing the floor work, following which stretches are performed.

Other considerations:
(1) *All participants should have an induction session, the purposes of which are:*
   ■ familiarization with each station and the equipment involved;
   ■ introduction to correct exercise technique;
   ■ determination of duration/intensity, etc., needed to achieve training heart rate;
   ■ individualization of prescription in the light of special needs, e.g. orthopaedic.
(2) *Staff/participant ratio must be sufficient to ensure:*
   ■ the handling of emergencies;
   ■ supervision of participants and opportunity to coach and correct technique;
   ■ monitoring of intensity levels (RPE, pulse monitoring, etc.).
(3) *Prior to each session participants should:*
   ■ have their heart rate and blood pressure checked;
   ■ be asked about new or changed symptoms;
   ■ be asked about changes in medication.

The Cardio-protective Diet

Eat:

- Skimmed/semi-skimmed milk
- Low fat yoghurts
- Virtually fat-free fromage frais
- Low-fat cheeses
- Cottage and curd cheese
- Low- or reduced-fat hard cheeses
- Low-fat cheese spreads
- Quark
- Medium-fat cheeses
- Edam, Brie, Camembert, Feta, Mozzarella, goat's cheeses
- Low- and medium-fat cheeses (no more than 200 g/8 ozs per week)
- Monounsaturated oils and margarines
- Polyunsaturated oils and margarines
- Low-fat spreads (in moderation)
- All white fish and oily fish
- Shellfish
- Chicken and turkey (skin removed)
- Game and rabbit
- Lean red meat, beef, veal, very lean pork or lamb; offal
- Soya protein meat substitutes
- Eggs (no more than 3–4 per week)
- Seeds, nuts and pulses
- Potatoes: jacket, boiled, mashed
- Wholewheat cereals, bread and flour; brown rice; wholewheat pasta; wholemeal currant buns; wholemeal scones
- Fresh fruit, salads and vegetables (at least five helpings per day)

Avoid:

- Whole gold top, Jersey, evaporated and condensed milk; skimmed milk with added vegetable fat
- Double, single, whipping, tinned or synthetic cream; cream substitutes, ice-cream, beverage whiteners
- High fat hard cheeses such as Stilton, Cheddar, processed cheese, cream cheese
- Butter, hard and soft margarines, lard, dripping, suet, solid vegetable oils, ghee, mayonnaise, salad cream
- Coconut and palm oil
- Fish in batter or breadcrumbs
- Goose and duck
- Fat on meat; sausages, salami, tinned meats, pâté, liver sausage, meat paste, black pudding, pork pies, sausage rolls
- Scotch eggs
- Chips, potato crisps
- Pastry, pastries, cakes, biscuits (unless home-made with suitable ingredients)
- Chocolate

Suitable cooking methods

- Grilling
- Steaming
- Casserole
- Boiling
- Poaching
- Barbecue
- Baking
- Microwave
- Stir-fry

Practical tips

Fat

Use as little oil and fat in cooking as possible. Choose ones high in MUFA or PUFA and always measure the amount of oil by the teaspoon rather than just pouring.

Oil

When using oil for deep frying (occasionally) do not re-use more than two or three times as the oil deteriorates and Vitamin E is destroyed.

Chips

Thinly cut chips have a much higher fat content than thick-cut chips. So if home-made, cut chips thickly and straight, fry in hot vegetable oil and blot with kitchen paper; or use reduced-fat oven chips.

Roasting

Cook roast potatoes in vegetable oil separately from the meat. Parboil potatoes and brush with suitable oil or dry roast.

Margarines

Spread chosen margarines or low-fat spreads thinly. Try sometimes to go without altogether especially if the topping is already moist, e.g. with beans (on toast), sardines (on toast), jam, etc.

Stir-frying

Stir-fry is an oriental way of cooking and relies on steaming rather than frying. Only small quantities of oil are necessary or oil and water/sherry and small, even sized vegetables, noodles, rice, fish, lean meat are stirred to cook quickly and evenly. Hot oil seals the food so that there is little uptake of fat and the food stays crisp.

Fish

Eat more fish, white or oily. White fish is low in total and saturated fat and two portions of oily fish should be eaten each week. Grill, microwave or bake rather than deep frying in batter. If fish is in breadcrumbs, bake or grill as breadcrumbs absorb large quantities of fat when fried.

Processed meats

Beefburgers and sausages are very fatty so don't use too often and choose low-fat varieties.

Nuts

Nuts are high in fat (except chestnuts) but do contain mostly MUFA (especially almonds and peanuts) and PUFA (especially walnuts) and are good sources of Vitamin E. Use for nut roasts and rissoles as an alternative to meat, use in muesli; nut butters, spread thinly, make suitable sandwich fillings.

Seeds

Seeds are nutritionally similar to nuts. Sesame, sunflower and pumpkin seeds can be added to muesli, crumble toppings, salads, cakes and nut dishes or eaten as seed spreads such as tahini.

Pulses

Pulses are peas, beans and lentils. They contain protein, are very low in fat, high in soluble fibre and a good source of iron – particularly important for non-meat eaters. They can be used on their own in vegetarian dishes or soups or used to extend meat meals. It is simple to add a tin of baked beans or peas to dishes. Beans can be bought ready cooked in tins or dried in packets. To cook dried beans, soak overnight and boil fast, uncovered, for ten minutes the next day, then reduce heat and cook beans until tender (cooking time depends on the bean). Cooked beans can be frozen for extra convenience.

Vegetables

Cook vegetables in the minimum amount of water, for the shortest period of time. Microwaving and steaming are excellent ways of cooking vegetables to retain the most nutrients. Vegetables should be served immediately as nutrient losses occur with keeping food warm. If vegetables are conventionally cooked the cooking water can be used for soups and stocks.

Take at least 5 – an example!

- fruit juice for breakfast
- two vegetables (plus potatoes) with the main meal (could include a side salad)
- salad in sandwiches or vegetable soup for a snack meal
- a fresh fruit as a pudding or snack.

Bread

Wholemeal and granary bread are nutritionally preferable to white bread as they contain more fibre and also vitamin E in the wheatgerm.

Oats

Oats contain soluble fibre which helps to reduce serum cholesterol and can be cooked as porridge, used as a base for muesli, and used with wholemeal flour for crumble toppings and coatings.

Salt

Enhance the flavour of food by using herbs, spices, pepper, mustard, lemon juice, vinegar and ginger instead of adding salt. Fresh, home-cooked food contains less salt than processed foods. Choose manufactured foods labelled with 'less salt added' or 'no salt added'. Salt substitutes are useful for some people who find giving up salt initially difficult. However, in time salt is tasted at lower concentrations and eventually substitutes may not be necessary.

Sugar

Sugar can be reduced by using naturally sweet fruits, fruit juices and dried fruits to sweeten foods, e.g.

- dried fruit or bananas added to breakfast cereals
- dried fruits, carrots, apples, bananas in cakes
- the use of low sugar in preserves, home-made or bought low sugar jams or the use of pure fruit spreads
- choose low-sugar products, diet squashes and carbonated drinks, low sugar jellies, etc.

Sugar substitutes: as with salt substitutes, these may be useful for helping people to give up sugar initially but in the long-term obtaining sweetness from sources with other available nutrients (e.g. anti-oxidants in fruit) is better nutritionally.

Appendix 6

Body Mass Index

Body Mass Index (BMI) is the most widely used method of classifying excess weight and can be calculated using the following formula:

$$\text{Body Mass Index (BMI)} = \frac{\text{Weight (kg)}}{\text{Height (m}^2)}$$

It is available in various forms of 'ready reckoner'. Garrow defines grades of weight as:

BMI		
	< 19	Underweight
	20–24.9	Acceptable weight
	25–29.9	Overweight
	30–39.9	Obese
	> 40	Severely obese

Reference

Garrow, J.S. (1981) *Treat Obesity Seriously*, Churchill Livingstone, Edinburgh.

Glossary

Adherence: degree to which individuals carry out the behaviours and treatments recommended to them by health professionals (also called **compliance**).

ATP (adenosine triphosphate): an energy rich compound which donates its energy to cell functions during its breakdown to ADP and Pi and accepts energy from the breakdown of food molecules during its formation from ADP and Pi.

Angina: pain in chest, neck, arm or jaw produced by lack of oxygen to the heart muscle (myocardium), not resulting in permanent damage.

Antioxidant: a substance that delays or prevents oxidation. Main dietary antioxidants are: vitamins E, C, A, beta carotene, and trace elements zinc, manganese, selenium and copper.

Body mass index (BMI): a classification of weight, calculated by weight (kg) divided by height (m^2).

Borg scale: a scale for rating perceived exertion developed by Gunnar Borg, in which the number 6 is associated with no exertion and the number 20 with maximal exertion. For practical purposes, ratings of perceived exertion measured with the Borg scale are considered reliable and valid estimates of effort (see **Rating of perceived exertion**).

Compliance: *see* **adherence**.

CR programme staff: any member of a multi-professional team whose remit includes direct contact with patients, or members of their family, who have access to a cardiac rehabilitation service.

CR participant: a patient who is participating in a cardiac rehabilitation programme.

Cardiac rehabilitation: a multi-factorial, multi-professional service, designed to cater for the needs of patients with coronary heart disease (and their families), with the objective of restoring them to as normal a life as possible.

Cholesterol: cholesterol is a fat-like, waxy material, present in the blood and most tissues in the body, especially nervous tissue. It is an essential component of cell membranes and a precursor of bile acids and steroid hormones.

Depression: a mood disorder whose main features are sadness and dejection, decreased motivation and interest in life, negative thoughts (such as feeling hopeless or low in self-esteem) and physical symptomatology (such as disturbed sleep, chronic fatigue, and loss of appetite and energy).

Dynamic exercise: alternate contraction and relaxation of a skeletal muscle or group of muscles, causing partial or complete movement through a joint's range of motion.

Endurance: the ability to sustain exercise at a high proportion of individual VO_{2max} or (in CHD patients) VO_{2peak} (see definitions).

Ergometer: an instrument used to measure work and power output.

Exercise prescription: a recommended regimen of physical activity which will enhance the health-related components of physical fitness and which varies in accordance with individual interests, habitual activity levels, age and health status.

Familial hypercholesterolaemia: an inherited condition which leads to very high concentrations of plasma cholesterol, usually in excess of 8.0 mmol/l. Associated with premature CHD and an accumulation of cholesterol deposits in tendons.

Fatty acids: polyunsaturated fatty acids which cannot be made in the body and need to be derived from linoleic and linolenic acids respectively.

Heart failure: syndrome in which reduced pumping capacity of the heart leads to shortness of breath, fatigue or oedema, at rest or on exertion.

High density lipoprotein: transport system which collects cholesterol from peripheral tissues and delivers it to the liver for elimination. High levels above 1.5 mmols/l are protective whilst low levels below 0.9 mmol/l confer a higher risk of CHD.

Isometric contraction: a type of muscular contraction in which there is no change in muscle length or movement of the skeleton.

Lipoprotein: lipids such as cholesterol and triglyceride are insoluble in water and therefore need to be transported in plasma bound to apolipoproteins. The resulting complexes are called lipoproteins and are classified according to their density.

Low density lipoprotein: a cholesterol-rich transport system which delivers cholesterol from the liver to peripheral tissues. LDL-cholesterol plays a causal role in atherosclerosis and a high level above 3.5 mmol/l, in the presence of other risk factors, confers a greater overall risk of CHD.

Maximal heart rate: the maximal number of times the heart contracts per minute; maximal heart rate is reduced with increasing age and average maximal values may be predicted by the equation 220 (beats per minute) minus age (years).

Metabolic equivalent unit (MET): a unit used to estimate the metabolic cost of physical activity; one MET equals oxygen consumption at rest, which is approximately 3.5 millilitres of oxygen per kilogram of body weight per minute ($3.5\,ml/kg^{-1}/min^{-1}$).

Meta-analysis: the name given to a set of techniques for reviewing research in which data from several primary studies are statistically combined.

Quality of life: a concept encompassing the broad range of physical and psychological characteristics and limitations which describe an individual's ability to function and derive satisfaction from doing so. Quality of life is now usually assessed from the perspective of the individual rather than as a rating by health or other professionals.

Rating of perceived exertion: quantification of the subjective intensity of physical effort (see **Borg scale**).

Respiratory exchange ratio (RER): the ratio of carbon dioxide produced to oxygen consumed.

Risk factor: factor known to increase the likelihood of future cardiac morbidity or mortality.

Risk stratification: a process whereby patients are grouped into levels of future risk (low, moderate, high), usually by a combination of assessment of risk factors and clinical status.

Self-efficacy: an individual's assessment of his or her competency to perform a particular behaviour successfully.

Sensitivity: the percentage of times that a test elicits an abnormal result when a diseased individual is tested.

Specificity: the percentage of times that a test elicits a normal result when a disease-free individual is tested.

Stress: the interaction between person and environment where the individual perceives that the demands being placed on him or her exceed his/her available resources and therefore threaten his/her well-being. The term is also used in exercise testing, which is sometimes referred to as 'stress-testing', relating to the physiological stress or load, rather than a psychological perception of stress.

Symptom-limited exercise test: an exercise test with progressive load until symptoms occur which the subject finds unacceptable, i.e. without a preset load or duration.

Thrombogenic: likely to cause or lead to thrombosis or clotting within a blood vessel.

Thrombolysis: a process whereby a clot is lysed, or dissolved. In heart attacks (myocardial infarction), a clot forming in a coronary artery can be thrombolysed using thrombolytic drugs (e.g. streptokinase), thereby dissolving the clot and restoring the blood supply to the heart muscle (myocardium).

Triglycerides: these constitute the major part of dietary fat. Each triglyceride is made up of a unit of glycerol and three fatty acids. These fatty acids differ with regard to their chain length, unsaturation, position and geometry (cis or trans) of their double bonds.

Trans fatty acids: hydrogenation (the industrial process of hardening oil used in the manufacture of margarines and shortenings) leads to the production of fatty acids with double bonds in the transconfiguration. These are referred to as trans fatty acids and are also found naturally in butter, beef and lamb. Most naturally occurring unsaturated fatty acids have their double bonds in the cis configuration.

Type A behaviour pattern: behaviour pattern associated with being rushed, competitive, very achievement-orientated and aggressive. Traditionally associated with higher risk of heart disease, although more recent evidence is equivocal.

VO_{2max}: maximal oxygen consumption.

VO_{2peak}: maximal oxygen consumption when maximal values attained are limited by presence of disease.

Useful Addresses

American Association of Cardiovascular and Pulmonary Rehabilitation

7611 Elmwood Avenue, Suite 201
Middleton
WI 53562
USA

Tel: 001 608 831 6989
Fax: 001 608 831 5122

Association of British Cardiac Nurses

Membership Secretary
Janet McKay
Level 4, East
Crosshouse Hospital
Kilmarnock
Ayrshire KE2 0BE

Tel: 01563 577693
Fax: 01563 577973

ASH (Action on Smoking and Health)

109 Gloucester Place
London, W1H 4EJ

Tel: 0171 935 3519
Fax: 0171 935 3463

British Association for Cardiac Rehabilitation

c/o Action Heart
Wellesley House
117 Wellington Rd
Dudley
West Midlands DY1 1UB

Tel: 01384 230222
Fax: 01384 254437

British Association of Counselling

1 Regent Place
Rugby
Warwickshire CV21 2PJ

Tel: 01788 550899
Fax: 01788 562189

British Association of Occupational Therapy

College of Occupational Therapy
6–8 Marshalsea Rd
Southwark
London SE1 1HL

Tel: 0171 357 6480
Fax: 0171 378 1353

British Cardiac Society

9 Fitzroy Square
London W1 5AH

Tel: 0171 383 3887
Fax: 0171 383 0903

British Heart Foundation

14 Fitzhardinge Street
London W1H 4DH

Tel: 0171 935 0185
Fax: 0171 486 1273

British Nutrition Foundation

52–54 High Holborn House
High Holborn
London WC1V 6RQ

Tel: 0171 404 6504
Fax: 0171 404 6747

British Psychological Society

St Andrew's House
48 Princess Rd East
Leicester LE1 7DR

Tel: 01533 549568
Fax: 01533 470787

Cardiac Rehabilitation Interest Group, Scotland

Physiotherapy Department
Stirling Royal Infirmary NHS Trust
Livilands
Stirling
FK8 2AU

Tel: 01786 434000
Fax: 01786 450588

Chartered Society of Physiotherapy

14 Bedford Row
London WC1R 4ED

Tel: 0171 242 1941
Fax: 0171 831 4509

Chest, Heart and Stroke Association (Northern Ireland)

21 Dublin Road   Tel: 01232 320184
Belfast BT2 7FJ   Fax: 01232 333487

Chest, Heart and Stroke Association (Scotland)

65 North Castle Street   Tel: 0131 225 6963
Edinburgh EH2 3LT   Fax: 0131 220 6313

Coronary Prevention Group

Plantation House, Suite 514 D + M   Tel: 0171 626 4844
31/35 Fenchurch Street   Fax: 0171 626 4748
London EC3M 3NN

European Association of Cardiovascular Rehabilitation

Patrick Van Daele   Tel: 00 32 15 506 135
EACVR Secretariat   Fax: 00 32 15 505 383
Centrum voor Cardiale Revalidatie
Imeldaziekenhuis v.z.w.
Imeldalaan 9-B 2820 Bonheiden
Belgium

Family Heart Association

7 High Street   Tel: 01865 370292
Kidlington   Fax: 01865 370295
Oxon OX5 2DH

Health Education Authority

Hamilton House   Tel: 0171 383 3833
Mabledon Place   Fax: 0171 387 0550
London WC1H 9TX

Heart Manual

Mary Ramsay, Co-ordinator   Tel: 0131 537 9127
BHF Research Unit   Fax: 0131 537 9120
Astley Ainslie Hospital
Grange Loan
Edinburgh EH9 2HL

Heart News (BHF)

BHF Heart News
The Gatehouse
112 Park Hill Road
Harborne
Birmingham
B17 9HD

Tel: 0121 428 4474
Fax: 0121 428 4474

Irish Heart Foundation

4 Clyde Road
Dublin 4
Ireland

Tel: 00 3531 668 5001
Fax: 00 3531 668 5896

Irish Association for Cardiac Rehabilitation

c/o Irish Heart Foundation (see above)

Look After Your Heart

64 Burgate
Canterbury
Kent CT1 2HJ

Tel: 01227 455564
Fax: 01227 458741

National Forum for Coronary Heart Disease Prevention

Hamilton House
Mabledon Place
London WC1H 9TX

Tel: 0171 383 7638
Fax: 0171 413 2638

Resuscitation Council (UK)

9 Fitzroy Square
London W1P 5AH

Tel: 0171 388 4678
Fax: 0171 383 0773

Royal College of Nursing

20 Cavendish Square
London W1M 0AB

Tel: 0171 409 3333
Fax: 0171 355 1379

Sports Council

16 Upper Woburn Place
London WC1H 0QP

Tel: 0171 388 1277
Fax: 0171 383 5740

St John's Ambulance Headquarters

1 Grosvenor Crescent
London SW1X 7EF

Tel: 0171 235 5231
Fax: 0171 235 0796

Index

BRITISH ASSOCIATION FOR CARDIAC REHABILITATION
MEMBERSHIP APPLICATION FORM

Please PRINT all information clearly:

FAMILY NAME: _____

FIRST NAMES: _____

TITLE: Prof Dr Mr Mrs Ms Miss Other _____

HOME ADDRESS: _____

_____

_____ POST CODE: _____

PLACE OF WORK: _____

ADDRESS: _____

_____

_____ POST CODE: _____

TELEPHONE: (Hm) Std: _____   No: _____

              (Wk) Std: _____   No: _____

              (Fax) Std: _____   No: _____

Please delete as applicable:

* I would prefer correspondence to be sent to my home address.

* I would prefer correspondence to be sent to my work address.

JOB TITLE: _____

EMPLOYER: _____

PROFESSIONAL QUALIFICATIONS   DATE

_____

_____

_____

_____

_____   PTO

AREAS OF EXPERTISE: (Please circle)

Risk factor assessment   Health Education
Management of hyperlipidaemia   Nutrition
Smoking cessation   Hypertension
Stress management   Psychological issues
Exercise prescription   Exercise testing
Vocational assessment   Counselling
Social work   Pharmacy
Programme management   Research

Please indicate your area(s) of experience of cardiac rehabilitation:

Phase 1   –   In-patient   Phase 2   –   First 4–6 weeks

Phase 3   –   Out-patient   Phase 4   –   Long term maintenance
                         programme incl
                         exercise

Please provide a brief description of your direct involvement in cardiac rehabilitation, <u>including</u> the number of hours/week:

_____

_____

_____

Any other comments: _____

_____

_____

I certify that the information provided in this application is correct and I agree to abide by the Association's Code of Ethics and Professional Conduct.

I enclose my membership fee:
Full membership (Health Professional)   –   *£25.00 per annum*
Individual Associate membership (Non Health Professional) £20.00 per annum
Student membership   –   *£12.50 per annum*

Please make cheques payable to B.A.C.R. and return completed form to B.A.C.R., c/o Action Heart, Wellesley House, 117 Wellington Road, Dudley, DY1 1UB.

Signature: _____ Date: _____